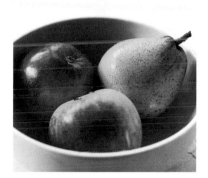

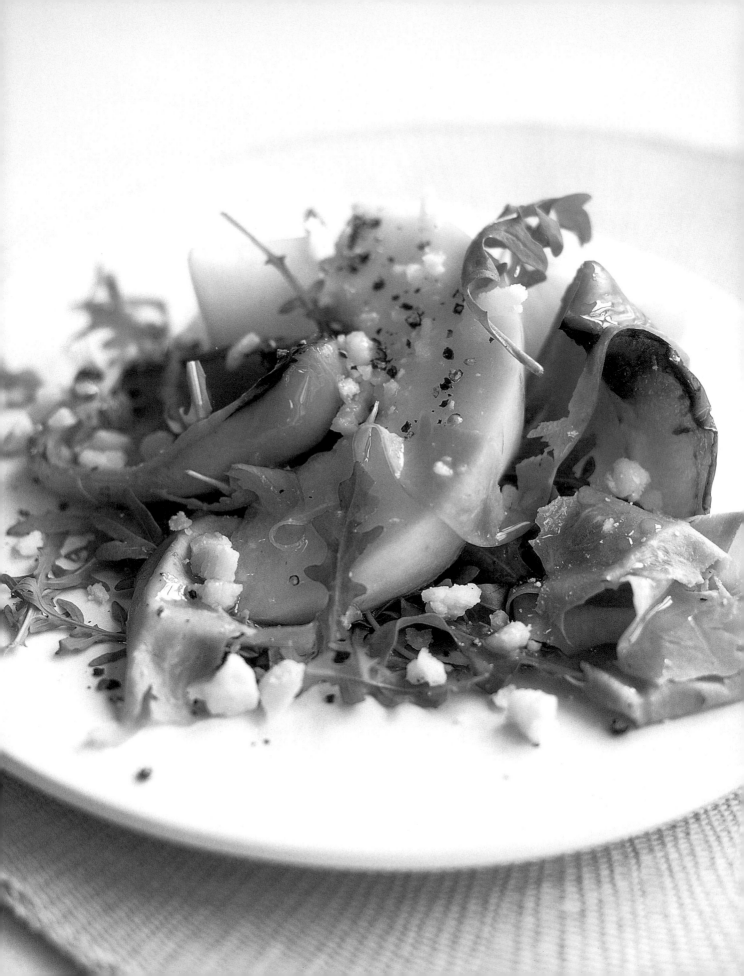

shortcuts to success

healthy

Lesley Waters

photography by Gus Filgate

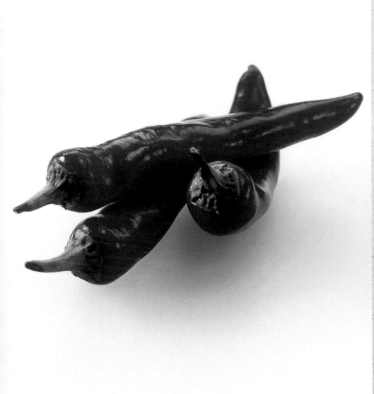

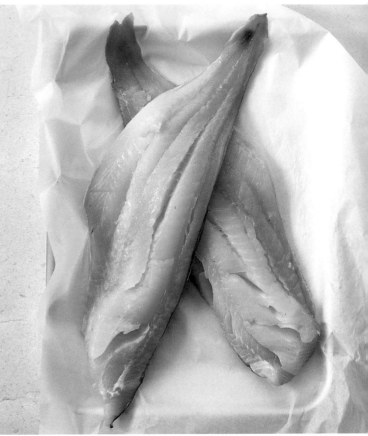

First published in the UK in 2003 by Quadrille Publishing Limited
Alhambra House 27-31 Charing Cross Road London WC2H OLS

This edition published by Silverback Books, Inc., San Fransisco, California. www.silverbackbooks.com
© in 2005

Editorial director Jane O'Shea **Creative director** Helen Lewis
Managing editor Janet Illsley **Art direction and design** Vanessa Courtier
Photographer Gus Filgate **Food stylist** Silvana Franco **Props stylist** Jane Campsie
Editors Barbara Croxford and Norma MacMillan **Production** Vincent Smith and Jane Rogers

Text © 2003 Lesley Waters Photography © 2003 Gus Filgate
Design and layout © 2003 Quadrille Publishing Limited

Cataloguing in Publication Data: a catalogue record for this book is available from the British Library.

ISBN 1 59637 013 0
Printed in China

contents

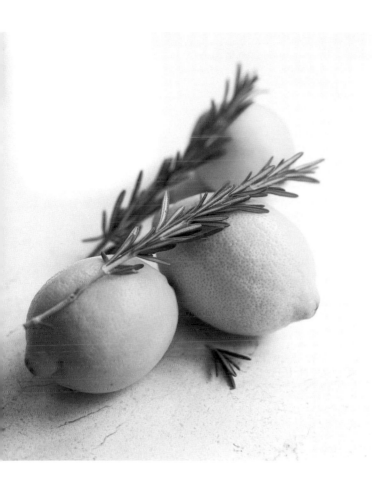

NOTES

Measurements are in standard American cups and spoons.

Use fresh herbs unless dried herbs are suggested.

Use freshly ground black pepper unless otherwise stated.

Eggs from cage-free or free-range hens are recommended, and extra large eggs should be used except where a different size is specified.

Recipes that feature raw or lightly cooked eggs should be avoided by vulnerable groups (anyone who is pregnant, babies and young children, the elderly, and those who are sick or who have compromised immune systems), unless using eggs that have been pasteurized in shell.

introduction

Whether I am working on television, teaching, or writing, I am often asked if it is really possible to deliver simple, tasty, healthy food every day, with a minimum of effort. And my answer is, yes, because for me this is what good food is all about. Healthy eating is not a fad, it's not a diet, nor is it something you practice for two weeks before your summer vacation. It's a great way to live and enjoy your food. And that, quite simply, is what this book is all about.

Most of us lead busy lives and time is precious. Finding the time to shop, cook, and eat three meals a day without resorting to quick fixes can seem impossible at times, but it can be done. Once hooked on a healthy diet, you will never look back and you will reap the benefits. I believe it is the simple changes that make the difference. It's not about giving up everything that is tasty and good to eat, just about making adjustments.

The key to healthy eating is about making changes that easily become part of your everyday life. One adjustment you can make is to invest in great fresh produce. Ask any top chef and he or she will tell you that to create tasty, simple food, quality is everything. Consider free-range and organic foods, and when it comes to fish and meat I look for the best quality possible, always bearing in mind that less is more and quality counts.

Enjoying your food in the company of others is a great way to socialize with family and friends, and helps children form good eating habits. However hectic your day is, do try to sit down to at least one meal with the family. Take the time to eat slowly and chew your food properly—this makes it easier to digest, and easier for your body to absorb the nutrients. Avoid overeating— recognize when you are full, then stop. Try not to skip meals, and you will really look forward to and enjoy the next meal.

This book begins with an introduction to the basic principles, or "building blocks," that are essential to a good diet. It covers balanced nutrition, judicious shopping, useful equipment, healthy cooking methods, and food safety. The recipe chapters that follow provide a wealth of exciting, tasty dishes, based on fresh ingredients and uncomplicated cooking techniques. Every meal occasion is covered, from breakfast, through lunchboxes and tasty snacks, to suppers and dinners. Scrumptious desserts are included too, because healthy eating is about a balanced approach to food, not excluding those foods that you enjoy.

For easy reference, the recipes are arranged according to the type of food: fish, chicken, and turkey, vegetables and salads, and so forth. Each recipe chapter contains an appropriate feature that includes several recipe ideas and healthy diet tips. With this innovative, easy-to-follow cookbook, you will soon find that healthy eating becomes a positive pleasure.

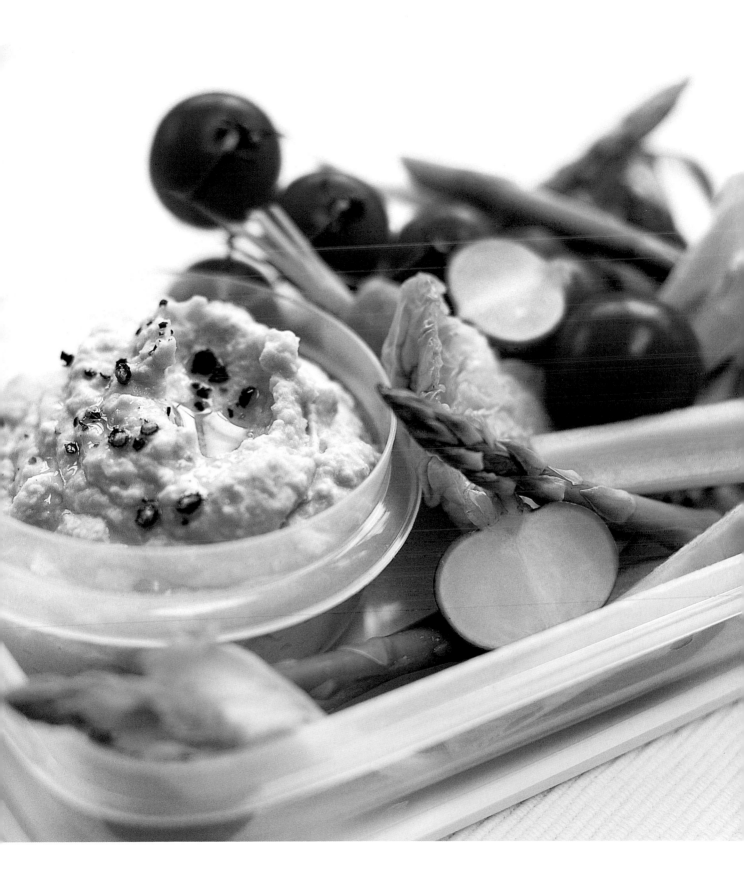

building blocks

Eating a variety of foods is the key to a nutritious, healthy diet. It's also important to balance your intake. The best diet includes plenty of fresh ingredients, covering the whole range of food types, to ensure your body gets enough of the essential nutrients: proteins, vitamins, minerals, carbohydrates, and fats. Some foods are obviously better than others—here is a guide.

Hydration

Our bodies are made up of approximately 80 percent water, so at the top of my list is water. Although it isn't a nutrient, water is vital for so many of our bodily functions. We should consume around 2 quarts (8 cups) of water a day. That is equivalent to 8 large glasses a day. For many of us, this is difficult to achieve, but other drinks help toward that target (excluding alcohol). And remember that many fruit and vegetables contain lots of water, so it all adds up. Tea and coffee both have a diuretic effect, encouraging the body to eliminate water, so they should be consumed in moderation. Always provide water with meals, and try to remember to drink at least a large glass or two in between meals.

Five-a-day fruit and veggies

This is the minimum recommended number of fruit and vegetable portions that we should consume every day. Fruit and vegetables are valuable because they supply the body's defence system with the vitamins, minerals, and fiber it needs to keep in good health. "Five-a-day" may seem a lot, but frozen and canned produce count too, as do dried fruits and fruit and vegetable juices.

Most vegetables and fruits are virtually fat-free and high in fiber, and they contain antioxidants, which boost the immune system and may help to protect the body from diseases, including some forms of cancer. Tomatoes, red bell peppers, mangoes, and avocados are particularly high in antioxidants. Vegetables and fruits vary in the essential nutrients they provide, so eat a good variety for maximum benefit. Fresh vegetables can be cooked in so many interesting ways, or eaten raw in salads or as crudités for dipping. Beyond the fruit bowl, enjoy quick smoothies, fruit salads, salsas, hot fruity desserts, and dried fruit as snacks. Buy good-quality fruit juice, or, if you have a juicer, make your own delicious vegetable and fruit juices.

Protein foods

We need far less protein than most of us consume—as little as 3 ounces of protein a day is generally sufficient. Again, variety is the key. White meat is a good source of protein and it has less saturated fat than red meat, although you can now buy very lean cuts of red meat. Fish is an excellent source of protein, especially oily fish such as salmon, mackerel, and sardines. And don't forget beans and lentils, nuts and seeds, which provide valuable vitamins and minerals too. Lastly, there is the versatile egg, a concentrated source of animal protein.

Salt

On average in this country, we consume about $1\frac{1}{2}$ times more salt than is recommended by health professionals. Too much salt can contribute to high blood pressure and has been linked to coronary heart disease, so it makes sense to cut down on your salt intake. These days, I do not use salt in my cooking.

If you wish to add salt to some of these recipes, that's fine, but try to cut down gradually. Perhaps the first step is to stop adding it during cooking. When you are accustomed to the new taste, banish the salt shaker from the table. It is amazing how quickly your taste buds adjust and you find you prefer less salt.

Sugar

Refined sugars provide "empty calories" and, if eaten frequently, increase the risk of tooth decay, so we should aim to cut down on consumption of these. Apart from the obvious sources, like candy, cookies, and cakes, watch out for hidden sugars in processed foods, such as sweetened breakfast cereals. Try to buy 'no added sugar' breakfast cereals and sweeten with naturally sweet fresh and dried fruits – try sprinkling raisins and fresh banana slices on muesli, for example.

Soft drinks, in particular, can contain large quantities of added sugar. Choose fresh fruit juices without added sugar, and look for lower sugar options if you buy fruit liqueurs.

Fats

In general, we consume too much fat. A small amount of fat plays an important part in the overall balance of a healthy diet, but eating too much can be harmful. Fats are composed of fatty acids, and it is the saturated type found in meat, dairy products, and hard cooking fats that are particularly harmful: A high intake of saturated fatty acids is linked to an increased risk of heart disease, obesity, and certain forms of cancer. To cut down, be wary of the hidden fats in bought cookies, cakes, pastries, and prepared meals. Opt for lean cuts of meat and smaller portions, filling your plate instead with plenty of vegetables. Choose strongly flavored cheese to use in cooking, such as Parmesan, because you need only a small amount for lots of taste. And butter? Well, it makes sense to cut down, but that doesn't mean you have to give it up. I prefer a fine scraping of butter on toast to any of the lower-fat spreads now available. It's all a question of awareness and a balanced approach.

Monounsaturated fatty acids are found in foods such as olive, sesame, and canola oils, avocados, seeds, and most nuts. These are not detrimental to health provided they are consumed in moderation, and they can help to lower cholesterol levels.

Polyunsaturated fatty acids include the essential omega-3 and omega-6 fatty acids that are important for growth, a healthy skin, and a strong immune system. Oily fish, soybeans, and canola oil are good sources of omega-3s; vegetable oils, such as sunflower, contain omega-6. These are beneficial sources of fat.

Hydrogenated fats found in margarine, shortening, and bought pastries and prepared meals, contain trans fatty acids that work like saturated fats. It is therefore preferable to avoid these or limit your intake in the same way as saturated fats.

Fiber

This isn't a nutrient as such, but it is an important constituent of food, which helps to keep the digestive system healthy. Wholegrain bread, cereals, fruit, vegetables, pulses and nuts are good sources.

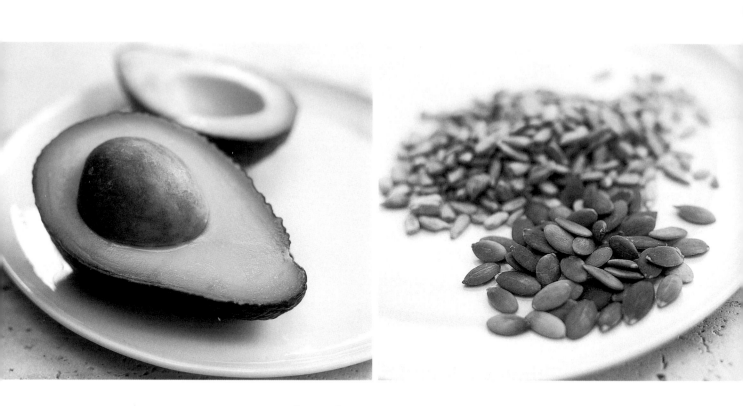

my top ten "super foods"

There are some foods that are so nutritious you could almost call them "super foods." These foods contain beneficial oils and/or high levels of antioxidants in the form of beta-carotene and vitamins C and E, all of which contribute to helping reduce the risk of serious diseases, such as heart disease and certain forms of cancer. Eat them regularly to maximize the benefits to your diet. Many foods could be described as "super foods," but these are my ten favorites.

Avocados   This fruit is rich in beneficial monounsaturated fatty acids, contains more protein than any other fruit, and is an excellent source of vitamin E.

Bananas   An excellent instant energy food and easy to digest, bananas are also high in potassium, magnesium and some B vitamins.

Berries   Black currants, blueberries, blackberries, and black grapes are all high in antioxidants.

Green vegetables   Brassicas, such as broccoli, Brussels sprouts, cabbage, and hearty greens, contain beneficial phytochemicals called indoles, which can help to detoxify the body when eaten regularly. They are also useful sources of minerals.

Oats   Wholegrain oats are an excellent source of soluble fiber and a slow-release form of carbohydrate. When eaten as part of a low-fat diet, oats can help to maintain a healthy heart.

Oily fish   All varieties—including salmon, mackerel, tuna, trout, and sardines—are good sources of protein and rich in beneficial omega-3 fatty acids, minerals, and certain vitamins.

Red and yellow bell peppers   Rich in beta-carotene and vitamin C.

Seeds   Sesame, pumpkin, and sunflower seeds are packed with protein, high in essential oils, and a valuable source of vitamin E and B vitamins.

Soy   An important high-quality vegetable protein food, especially for vegetarians, soy is also a good source of minerals, B vitamins, and antioxidants. It can be bought as bean curd (tofu), and soy milk, cheese, and yogurt.

Tomatoes   Another colorful food that is rich in beta-carotene and a good source of vitamins C and E.

"pantry" essentials

Certain ingredients have become the jewels of my kitchen cupboards, refrigerator, and freezer. These items ensure that tasty, healthy meals are achievable every day. I would be lost without them. In addition, I always have lots of apples, pears, oranges, lemons and limes, and bananas.

"Pantry"   Here, I keep a selection of the basic grain staples such as pasta, couscous, bulgur wheat, cornmeal, and different rices, plus different colored lentils, canned beans and tomatoes, and packages of nuts and seeds. For flavoring dishes, my pantry jewels are: Thai curry pastes, coconut milk (preferably reduced-fat), wine and balsamic vinegars, soy, teriyaki, Tabasco, and Worcestershire sauces, Dijon and grain mustards, dried chili flakes, and a selection of spices including ground coriander, sweet paprika, and garam masala. If you are trying to cut down on salt, these flavorings—together with fresh herbs, ginger, and garlic—will give you all the taste you need. You'll also need good-quality olive oil to use in moderation for cooking and salad dressings. And for flavoring sweet dishes, you'll find honey, maple syrup, and vanilla extract invaluable.

Refrigerator   Here, there is always fresh fruit juice, milk, yogurt, eggs, a piece of sharp cheddar, and a wedge of Parmesan. Lean bacon, olive tapenade, tahini, and fresh pesto sauce are there to add flavor to simple staples. In the vegetable drawer, you'll find nutritious broccoli, carrots, bell peppers, and baby spinach leaves. The salad crisper invariably contains a bag of salad leaves, ripe red tomatoes, cucumber, and a selection of chili peppers for easy raitas and spicy salsa.

Freezer   I have never been inclined to cook up meals for the freezer. They lose some qualities on freezing and I prefer to eat dishes at their best. However, I would not be without my freezer standbys, such as corn kernels, peas, and spinach, red summer fruits, and frozen yogurts. A few pita breads and good-quality loaves are always handy for those occasions when you run short.

key cooking methods

Modern cooking equipment greatly increases the options for healthy cooking techniques. Good-quality nonstick pans enable you to create appetizing, tasty dishes using the minimum of fat. They are important for many of the recipes in this book and essential for methods such as steam-frying. If you do not have them already, invest in a large nonstick wok with a lid, a shallow nonstick frying pan with a lid, one or two nonstick saucepans, and nonstick roasting pans. For baking, nonstick muffins pans and good-quality nonstick baking sheets make all the difference.

Steaming

Steaming is a classic cooking method for healthy food. Chinese bamboo steamers are an attractive option that can be used for serving the food as well as cooking it. Alternatively, try a metal fan-style steamer that opens out to fit the pan, or a special purpose pan with a perforated steamer that fits snugly on top or inside. A tight-fitting lid is essential to trap in the steam. Bring the water to a boil in the base pan, then put the food in the steamer and cover tightly. The food cooks in the trapped steam and most of the water-soluble vitamins and minerals are retained. You will need to check the water level every so often, to make sure the pan doesn't boil dry.

Poaching

Poaching is an ideal way to cook delicate foods that are inclined to break easily, such as eggs and fish. Bring the liquid to a boil in the pan, then lower the heat and wait until the surface is barely trembling before you add the food. Poaching is also a good method for foods that are liable to become dry. Chicken breasts, for example, remain succulent if you poach them gently in stock or wine flavored with herbs, and you can use the poaching liquor to make a tasty sauce.

Pan-grilling

Traditional cast-iron grill pans are heavy to use, and while they may be great for cooking steaks and chops, they are not much good for cooking anything else. The modern, lightweight, nonstick grill pan is ideal for cooking meat, fish, vegetables, and fruits, even for toasting bread. Pan-grilling is like upside-down broiling, or indoor grilling: the heat of the pan sears the food on the outside, giving it an inviting appearance, taste, and texture. There's the added advantage that very little fat is needed. Make sure the grill pan is really hot before you start. If you need a little oil, this should be brushed onto the food, not the pan. Press down on the food with the back of a turner or slotted spatula as it cooks, to give well-defined grill lines, but don't move it around too much.

Stir-frying

The Asian art of stir-frying is a fast, healthy way of cooking food, and nutrients are well retained. Once again you need to start with a hot pan, but this time when the food is added, you need to keep it moving to ensure even cooking. Have all your ingredients ready, chopped or sliced to a similar size before you start—once you start you can't stop! Make sure the wok is really hot before you add any ingredients, and avoid adding too many items at once, otherwise you will lower the temperature. Use a large spoon, wooden spatula, or turner to toss and stir the food constantly.

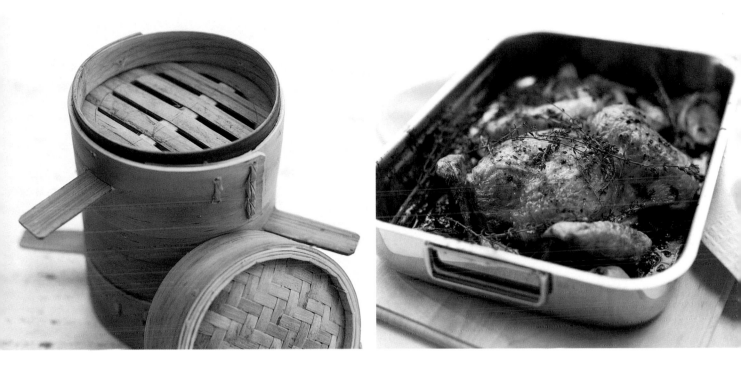

Steam-frying

I learned this brilliant way of cooking from a good friend. It is a simple technique that uses the minimum amount of oil, while maximizing the flavors in the food. Using a nonstick pan, start to fry the ingredient(s) in a little oil over a medium heat until slightly colored. Add a tablespoon or so of water and cover immediately with a tight-fitting lid to create steam in the pan. Continue to cook over a low heat. If your lid isn't really tight, cover the food directly with a damp piece of parchment paper and then with a lid. Don't keep lifting the lid, because steam will be lost and the pan will dry out. Should this happen, just add a splash more water.

Broiling

Meat, fish, and vegetables can all benefit from broiling, as it sears the outside of the food, leaving it juicy and succulent within. Preheat the broiler, and keep a close eye on the food as it cooks, turning frequently to ensure even cooking. If it appears to be browning too quickly, move the shelf down so the food is farther from the heat.

Roasting

This familiar cooking method requires the least effort on the part of the cook. Simply preheat the oven to the right temperature, toss the foods in a roasting pan with a little oil or marinade, and place in the oven. The dry heat draws out the juices from the food, concentrating the flavors, and browning the surface to delicious effect. You will probably need to turn or baste the food occasionally during roasting, but do this out of the oven, remembering to shut the oven door meanwhile, to keep the oven temperature up.

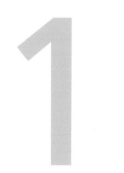

breakfasts, snacks, and packed lunches

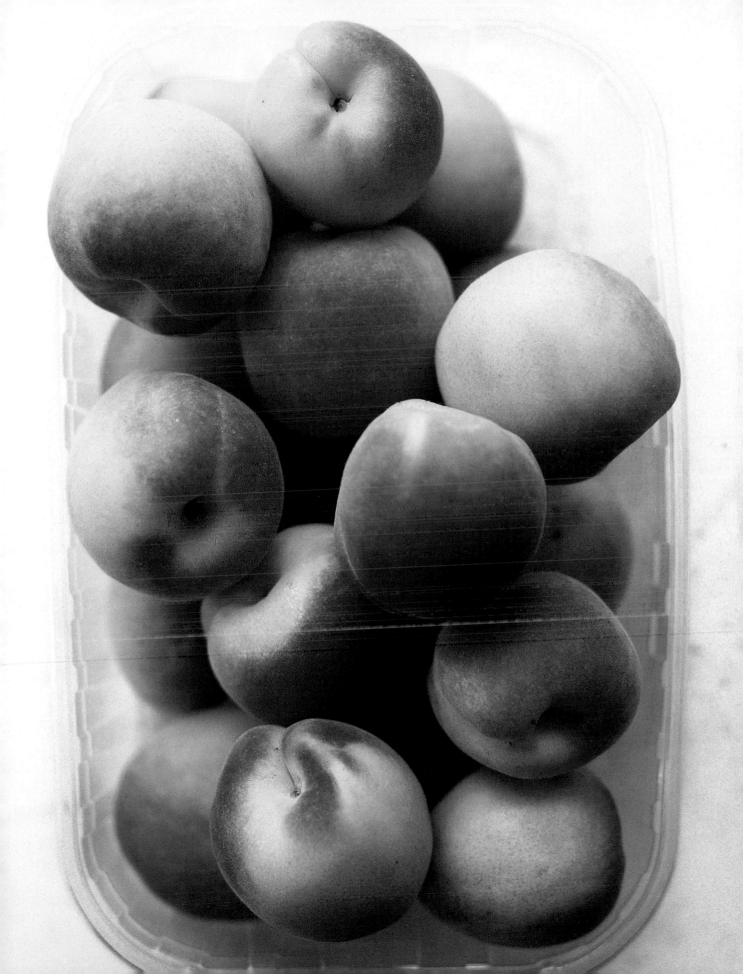

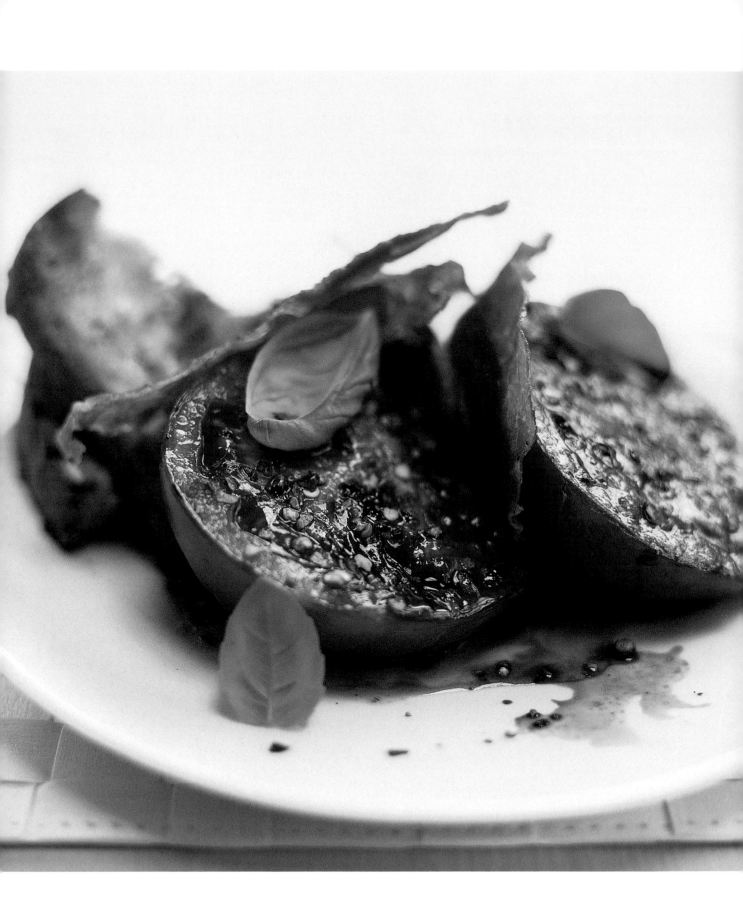

spiked balsamic tomatoes with crisp ham

Breakfast with a zing—sizzling tomatoes with an extra bite of chili and piquant balsamic vinegar to get you started. If you don't fancy chili in the morning, try scattering a little shredded fresh basil over the tomatoes instead, or omit the balsamic vinegar and sprinkle with the more traditional Worcestershire sauce. Tomatoes are a great source of vitamins A and C.

SERVES 4

4 beefsteak tomatoes, halved
1 teaspoon dried chili flakes
1 teaspoon sugar
1½ tablespoons olive oil
3 oz prosciutto or Black Forest ham
balsamic vinegar, for drizzling
freshly ground black pepper
basil leaves, for serving (optional)

1 Preheat the oven to 400°F. Place the tomatoes, cut-side up, on a nonstick baking sheet. Mix together the chili flakes, sugar, and olive oil, then drizzle this over the tomato halves. Grind plenty of black pepper over the top. Bake for 12–15 minutes until the tomatoes are cooked through and hot but still keeping their shape.

2 Meanwhile, broil the ham for 1 minute each side or until crisp. Place the tomatoes on four warm serving plates, then drizzle each with a little balsamic vinegar. Top with the crisp ham, scatter on some basil leaves, if you like, and serve, with wholegrain toast.

apricot and maple muffins

Even with added fiber-rich bran, these fruity muffins remain beautifully moist. They are flavored with dried apricots, one of the best sources of iron and potassium, and sweetened with maple syrup. Great for breakfast on the go, or simply pack them into lunchboxes.

MAKES 10

2 eggs
1 cup lowfat milk
2 tablespoons olive oil
3 tablespoons plain yogurt
1^1/$_2$ cups All-bran

1^2/$_3$ cups all-purpose flour
1 tablespoon baking powder
2 tablespoons light brown sugar
1 cup chopped dried apricots
^{1}/$_3$ cup golden raisins
2 tablespoons maple syrup

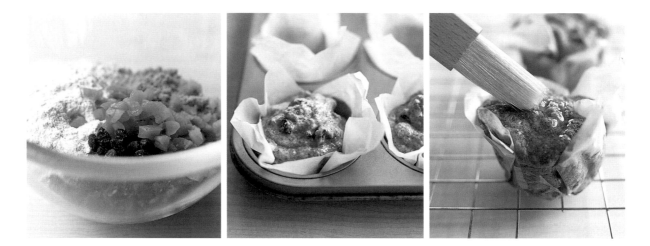

1 Preheat the oven to 375°F. Line 10 cups of a large muffin pan with muffin cases or wax paper. Mix together the eggs, milk, olive oil, yogurt, and bran. Set aside.

2 Sift the flour and baking powder into a bowl, then stir in the sugar, dried apricots, and raisins. Add the egg mixture and stir until evenly combined. Spoon the mixture into the muffin cases.

3 Bake for 15–20 minutes until golden and cooked through. Insert a skewer into the middle of one muffin to test—when done, the skewer will come out clean. Remove from the oven.

4 Let the muffins cool in the pan for a couple of minutes, then transfer to a wire rack and brush with the maple syrup. Serve warm or at room temperature.

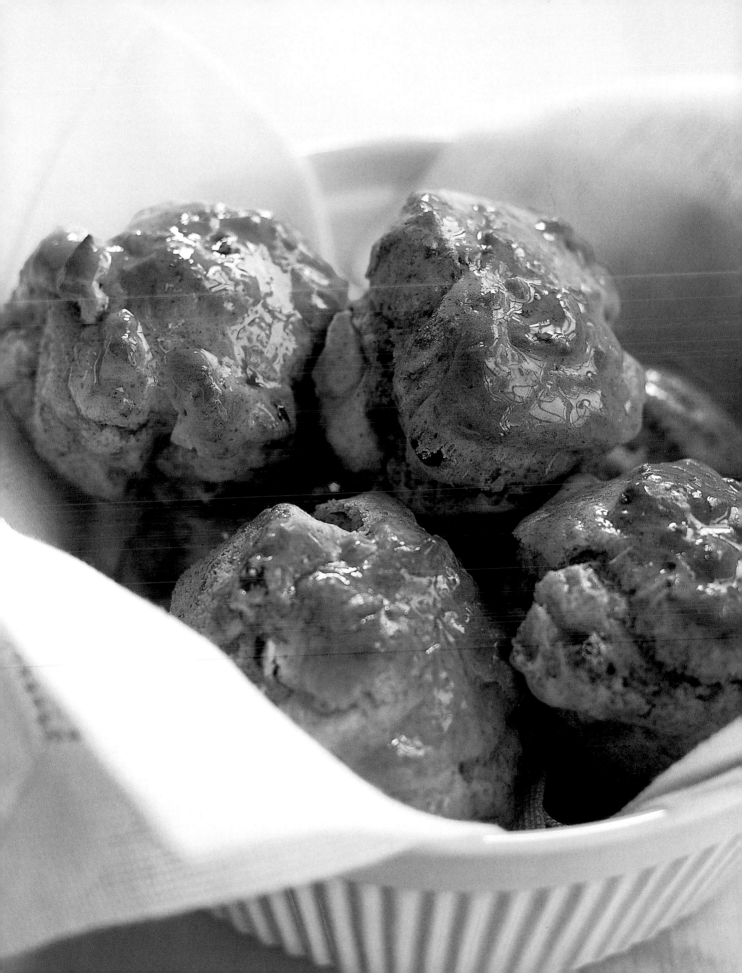

banana breakfast bread

A simple, quick bread that oozes with hot honeyed bananas. Bananas are a good source of vitamin B6, which is said to fight off viruses, plus vitamin C and magnesium. They're an ideal fruit to eat between meals, to give you that energy burst you sometimes need during the day.

MAKES 9 LARGE ROLLS

8-oz package pizza dough mix
3 medium bananas, peeled
grated zest of 1 orange
1 tablespoon poppy seeds
1/2 teaspoon ground cinnamon
1 1/2 tablespoons honey

1   Preheat the oven to 400°F. Lightly oil an 8-inch square nonstick baking pan. Make up the dough according to the package directions. Roll out to a rectangle, approximately 12 x 10 inches.

2   Slice the bananas and place in a bowl with the orange zest, poppy seeds, cinnamon, and half of the honey. Toss to mix, then spoon the mixture over the dough, leaving a 1/2-inch border.

3   Roll up the dough from a long side and press the edges together to seal. Cut across into nine equal pieces and place the pieces, cut-side up, in the pan.

4   Bake for 15–20 minutes. Warm the remaining honey in the microwave for 5 seconds (or in a small pan) and brush over the breakfast bread. Leave to cool slightly in the tin, then remove. Pull the rolls apart to serve. Best served warm.

tea-scented warm fruits

This simple dried fruit compote is perfect served with oatmeal or breakfast wheat flakes, or simply on its own. As well as being full of fiber, dried fruits are a good source of iron. Other varieties can be substituted, such as dried apricots.

SERVES 4
1 cup dried figs
1 cup prunes
1 cup dried pears
2 lemon-flavored green tea bags
1 tablespoon honey

1 Put the dried figs, prunes, and pears into a saucepan. Add the tea bags, 2½ cups water, and the honey. Bring to a boil, then lower the heat and simmer for 10 minutes.

2 Remove the tea bags, and tip the fruits and syrup into a non-metallic bowl. Serve warm, or let cool, then cover and refrigerate until needed.

oaty orange and fig pots

There's nothing like oats to set you up for the day. Oats are good for your heart, as they help reduce cholesterol, and they encourage the digestive system to run smoothly. Here, orange juice and chopped figs provide an added kick of vitamin C and fiber.

SERVES 2
1½ cups large rolled oats
4 dried figs, roughly chopped, or a large
  handful of raisins
1¼ cups orange juice
FOR SERVING:
thick plain yogurt
toasted sliced almonds (optional)

1 Divide the oats and figs between two serving bowls and pour the orange juice over. Cover and chill for 4 hours or overnight.

2 To serve, top each portion with a spoonful of yogurt and sprinkle with toasted almonds, if desired.

a healthy start

Breakfast is a meal that is often ignored, overlooked, or deliberately skipped, either through lack of time or interest, or in the mistaken belief that it will help with weight loss. In fact, a tasty breakfast will set you up for the day, getting your body working better and your brain moving faster. Slow-release carbohydrates, like oats and bran, are perfect for keeping you going through a busy day, so you won't start to feel hungry mid-morning.

If you are a really rushed household at the start of a day, breakfast in a glass may be more suited to your weekday mornings. For the earlier risers, pancakes or eggs might just tempt you to the table (these are great on weekends, too). Either way, it doesn't have to be a huge meal, just a tasty plate, bowl, or glassful to give you the best start to the day. Set your alarm in time—you'll be glad you did! Each of the following healthy breakfasts serves 4.

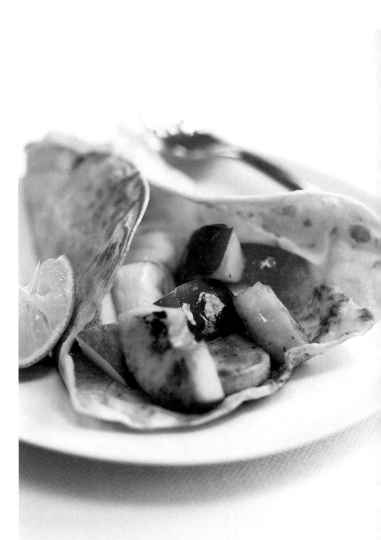

toasted breakfast wraps

Chop 2 large bananas and 2 nectarines; toss with 2 tsp honey. Heat a nonstick grill pan over a medium heat. Spoon the fruit down the center of 4 flour tortillas and roll up, folding in the ends neatly. Place seam-side down in the pan. Cook for 2 minutes each side. Serve warm.

Alternatively, fill tortillas with scrambled eggs made with 4 eggs, 1 cup shredded cooked ham, and a handful of cherry tomatoes, halved. Cook as above.

posh oatmeal

Make oatmeal according to the package directions, using half lowfat milk and half water. Top with a spoonful of plain yogurt, plus some chopped dried figs and toasted sliced almonds. For a refreshing summer option, top the oatmeal with blueberries and a drizzle of maple syrup.

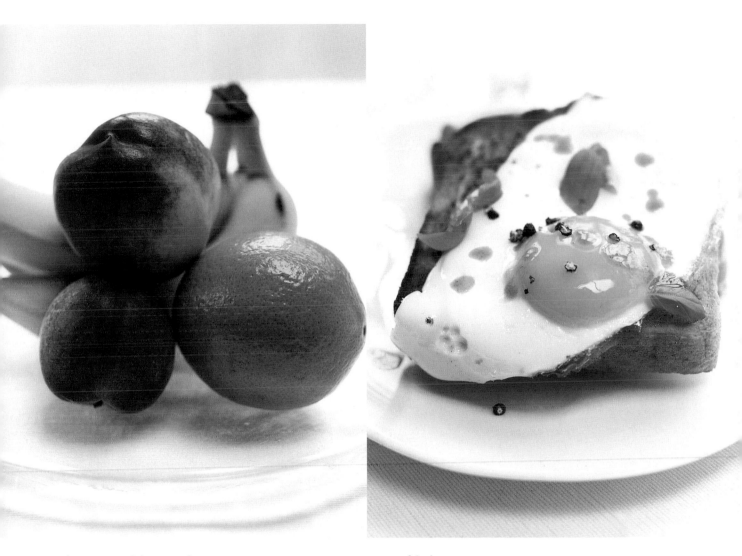

cinnamon-raisin pancakes

Sift ¾ cup self-rising flour and ½ tsp ground cinnamon into a bowl. Stir in 1½ tbsp sugar, the grated zest of 1 orange, and ⅓ cup golden raisins. Make a well in the center. Beat 1 egg with scant 1 cup milk and pour into the well. Stir to combine and form a smooth batter. Stir in 1½ cups crumbled bran flakes. Heat a large nonstick frying pan. Drop tablespoonfuls of the batter into the pan, spacing them apart, and cook for 2 minutes each side until set and golden. Serve warm.

steam-fried eggs

Heat a large, nonstick frying pan until very hot, then carefully wipe with a paper towel dipped in olive oil. Break 4 eggs into the pan and reduce the heat to low. Cover, so they start to steam, and cook for about 4 minutes for soft yolks; flip over for a firm set yolk. Season with black pepper, scatter a little torn basil over, and serve on hot toast. For a spicy variation, flavor with a dash of green Tabasco sauce and scatter on torn cilantro instead of basil.

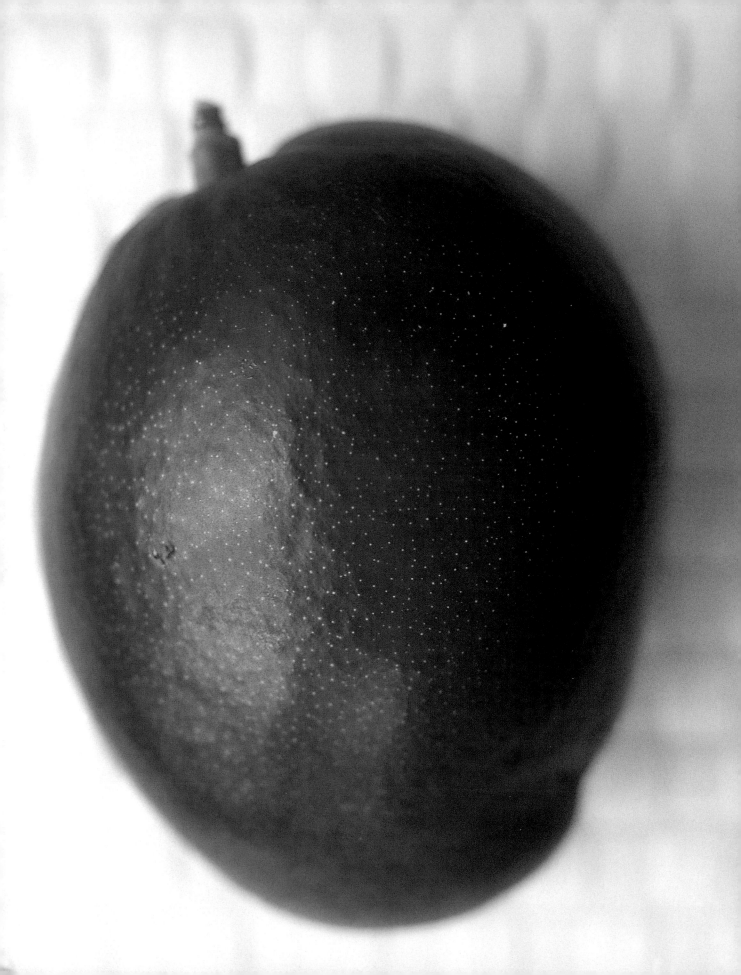

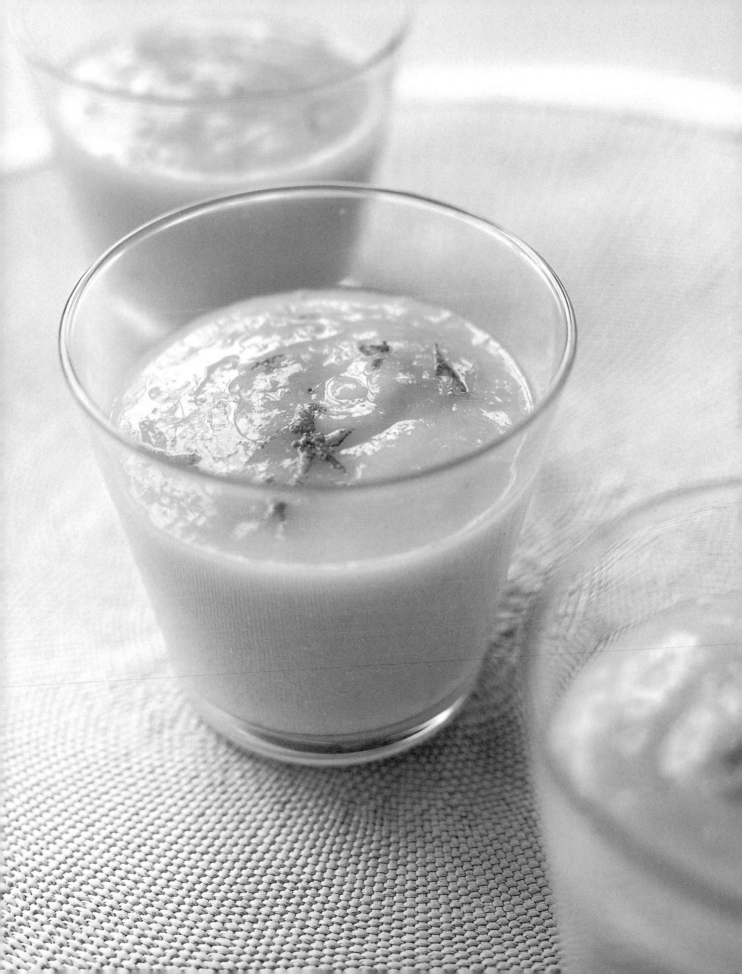

mango and banana smoothie

A healthy drink is a great start to the morning, and with a smoothie you can increase your fruit and fiber intake at the flick of a switch! Make sure the fruit is really ripe, otherwise the consistency and natural sweetness won't be quite right. *Illustrated on page 25*

SERVES 2–4

1 large, ripe banana, peeled and chopped
1 large, ripe mango, peeled and flesh sliced
  away from central seed

grated zest and juice of 1 lime
1 cup orange juice, or more to taste

1 Place the banana, mango, lime zest and juice, and orange juice in a blender. Blend until smooth, adding more orange juice if required to obtain the desired consistency. Pour into two large glasses or several smaller ones and serve right away.

pineapple and passion slush

Creamy and refreshing in one hit—a great start to the morning, or to enjoy at any time as one of your five-a-day fruit and veggies. Be sure to buy pineapple canned in its own juice, rather than heavy syrup.

SERVES 4

15 oz canned pineapple slices, in natural juice

1¼ cups plain nonfat yogurt
1 passion fruit, halved

1 Place the pineapple slices and juice in a blender with the yogurt. Put 10 ice cubes into a plastic bag and bash with a rolling pin to crush lightly. Tip the ice into the blender and whiz until frothy and just smooth. Pour the drink into four glasses and spoon a little passion fruit pulp on top to serve.

pink panther

This delicious drink provides a real burst of energy in a glass and boosts your vitamin C intake. For a summer cooler, replace the vanilla yogurt with vanilla frozen yogurt.

SERVES 2–4

1½ cups mixed strawberries and raspberries

⅔ cup cranberry juice
1 cup vanilla-flavored low-fat yogurt

1 Place the strawberries, raspberries, cranberry juice, and vanilla yogurt in a blender, and whiz until smooth. Fill two large glasses or several smaller tumblers with crushed ice and pour in the drink.

chunky pear and vanilla bars

These crumbly, fruity oat bars are high in fiber and low in fat. Packed with cranberries and pears, they make a great lunchbox-filler, or snack at any time of the day. Buy pure vanilla extract rather than vanilla flavoring—it has a far superior flavor.

MAKES 10

7 tablespoons honey
1 tablespoon vanilla extract
2 cups rolled oats
1/2 cup dried cranberries
2 small, ripe pears, peeled, cored, and chopped

1 Preheat the oven to 350°F. Heat the honey in a saucepan, then add the vanilla and stir in the oats, cranberries, and pears.

2 Press the mixture into a 7-inch square nonstick baking pan. Bake for 20 minutes. Let cool in the pan for 10 minutes, then mark into 10 bars and let cool completely.

raisin and cranberry rockies

These quick and easy, sustaining treats are best eaten on the day they are made. Dried cranberries lend a tangy, sweet flavor.

MAKES 8

2 tablespoons unsalted butter
3/4 cup self-rising flour
3 tablespoons brown sugar
2 tablespoons golden raisins
3 tablespoons dried cranberries
1 egg, beaten
1 tablespoon milk

1 Preheat the oven to 350°F. Lightly oil a nonstick baking sheet. Put the butter and flour into a mixing bowl and rub together with your fingertips until the mixture forms fine crumbs. Stir in the sugar, raisins, and cranberries. Mix in the egg and milk to form a soft dough.

2 Drop spoonfuls of the dough onto the baking sheet, spacing out well. Bake for 12–15 minutes until golden. Transfer to a wire rack to cool.

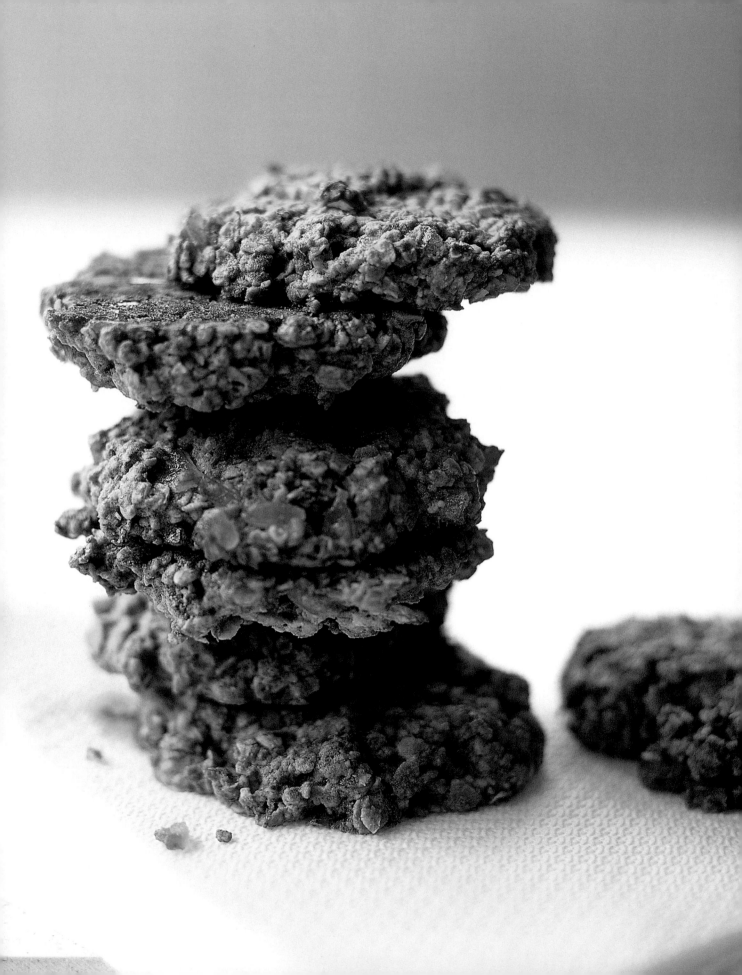

mango and carrot crumble cookies

Crumbly around the edges and moist in the middle, these cookies are a great favorite with my children. The grated fresh carrot and dried mango lend sweetness and plenty of goodness. Rolled oats provide crunch and soluble fiber, which, when eaten as part of a lowfat diet, can help maintain a healthy heart.

MAKES 16

4 tablespoons butter

1/3 cup packed dark brown sugar

1 egg

1/3 cup all-purpose flour

1/2 teaspoon baking soda

2 cups rolled oats

1 small carrot, peeled and grated

1/2 cup finely chopped dried mango

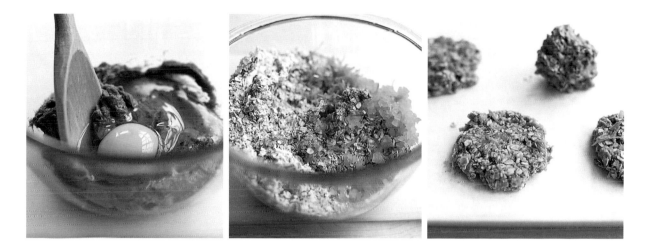

1 Preheat the oven to 375°F. In a large bowl, cream the butter and sugar together. Add the egg and beat until well mixed.

2 Add the flour, baking soda, rolled oats, grated carrot, and chopped mango to the mixture. Fold in, using a large metal spoon, until evenly mixed.

3 Drop tablespoons of the dough onto a nonstick baking sheet and press down gently. Bake for 15–20 minutes or until lightly golden around the edges.

4 Leave the cookies on the baking sheet for a few minutes, then transfer to a wire rack to cool.

houmous

This really creamy, protein-rich houmous is so easy to make. Provide a colorful selection of vegetables for dipping, such as carrot and celery sticks, cherry tomatoes, crunchy radishes, and little lettuce hearts. There's no need to cook dried chick peas—canned chick peas are perfect for this. Tahini is a thick paste made from sesame seeds, which provide the body with calcium, good for strong bones and teeth.

SERVES 4

14 oz canned chick peas (garbanzo beans),
  drained and rinsed
14 oz canned lima beans, drained and rinsed
2 garlic cloves, peeled and crushed
2 tablespoons tahini
3 tablespoons extra virgin olive oil
3 tablespoons plain yogurt
juice of 1/2 lemon
sea salt and freshly ground black pepper

1 Put the chick peas, lima beans, garlic, tahini, olive oil, yogurt, and lemon juice in a food processor and add about 5 tablespoons cold water. Blend until just smooth.

2 Season the houmous with a little sea salt and pepper to taste. Transfer to a bowl or plastic tub and serve with vegetable dippers and pita bread strips.

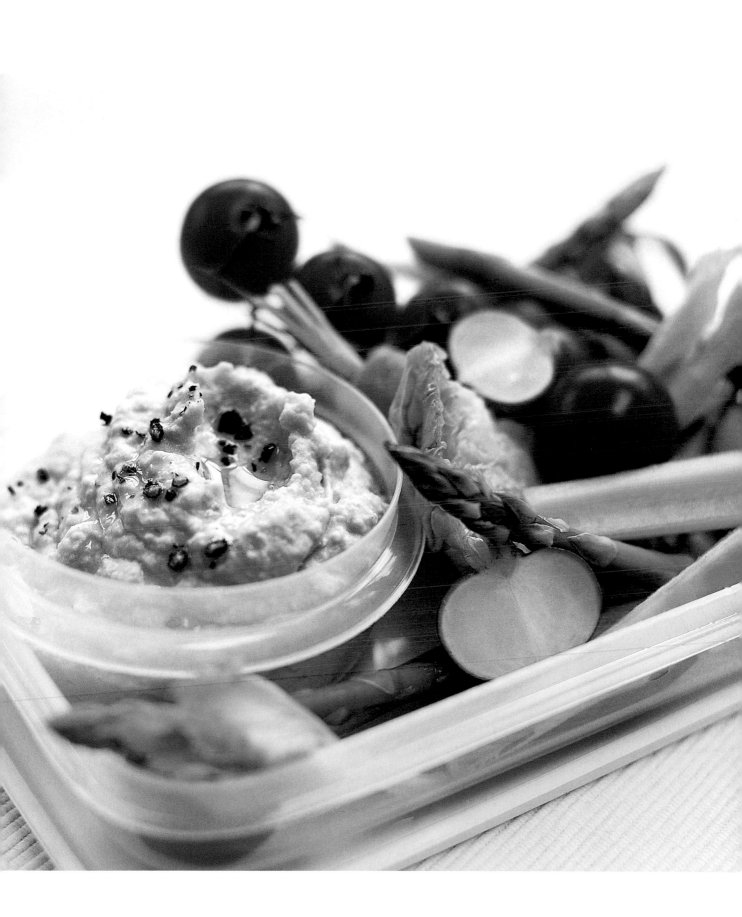

tuna pan bagna

This is a crusty roll filled to the brim with juicy sun-dried tomatoes, crisp leaves, tuna, and a creamy dressing. Canned tuna is high in protein and vitamins, but unfortunately it is not a good source of the omega-3 essential fatty acids, which are found in the fresh fish, because most of these are lost in the canning process.

MAKES 4

4 crusty bread rolls
6 tablespoons plain yogurt
1 garlic clove, peeled and crushed
1 teaspoon lemon juice
1/2 cup sun-dried tomatoes packed in oil,
  drained and chopped
crisp salad leaves
14 oz canned white-meat tuna in water,
  drained
freshly ground black pepper

1 Cut the top off each roll to make a lid. Hollow out the center of the rolls. (Use the bread that you remove to make crumbs and freeze until needed.)

2 To make the dressing, whisk the yogurt, garlic, and lemon juice together in a bowl, then season with pepper to taste.

3 Spoon the tomatoes into the cavities in the rolls and cover with a layer of salad leaves. Spoon on some of the yogurt dressing, then add the tuna, more dressing, and a few more salad leaves, pressing down lightly as you fill the rolls.

4 Place the lids on top to enclose the filling and press lightly. Wrap the rolls in wax paper and refrigerate or keep in a chilled insulated lunchbox for a few hours before eating (no longer or they may become a little soggy).

pesto picnic pasta

This nutritious salad is ideal to pack in lunchboxes. The pasta soaks up all the lovely flavors of the basil pesto and marries well with tender chicken, juicy tomatoes, and cucumber.

SERVES 4–6

7 oz pasta shapes, such as penne or shells

3 tablespoons pesto sauce

2 tablespoons extra virgin olive oil

1 heaped cup shredded cooked chicken breast

8 oz cherry tomatoes, halved

1 hothouse cucumber, peeled, seeded, and chopped

freshly ground black pepper

1 Cook the pasta in a large pan of boiling water, according to package directions, until *al dente* (tender but firm to the bite). Drain and rinse under cold water to stop further cooking, then place in a large bowl and set aside to cool completely.

2 Meanwhile, for the dressing, whisk the pesto and olive oil together in a large mixing bowl. Season with pepper.

3 Add the pasta, chicken, tomatoes, and cucumber to the pesto dressing and toss well together. Transfer the pasta salad to a container, cover, and store in the refrigerator until needed.

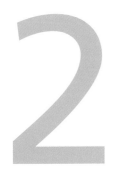

2 soups

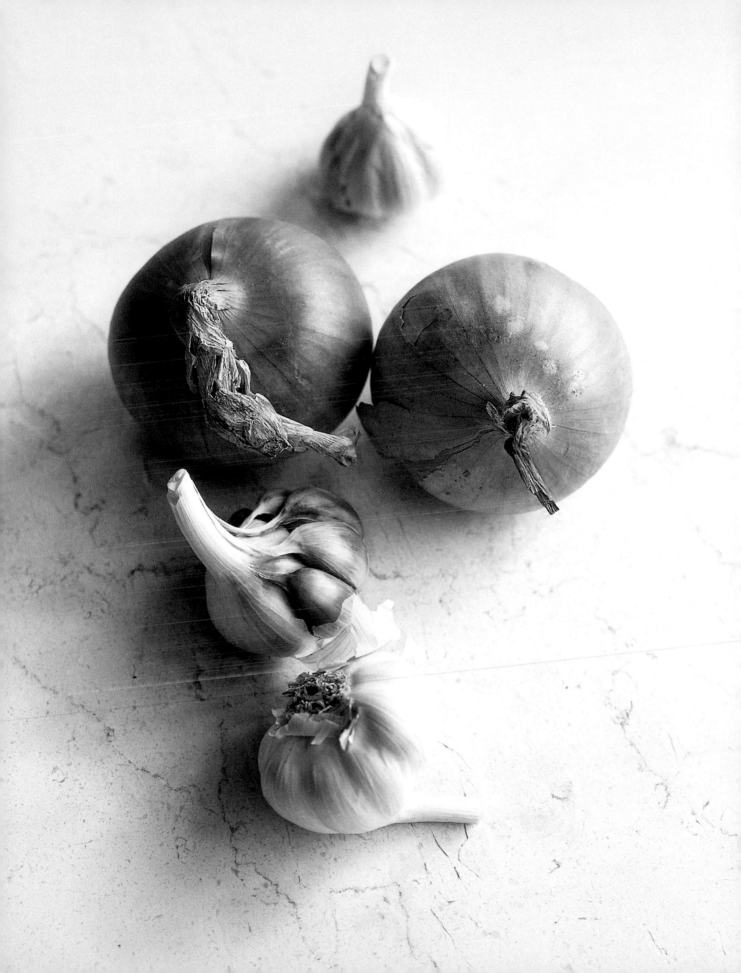

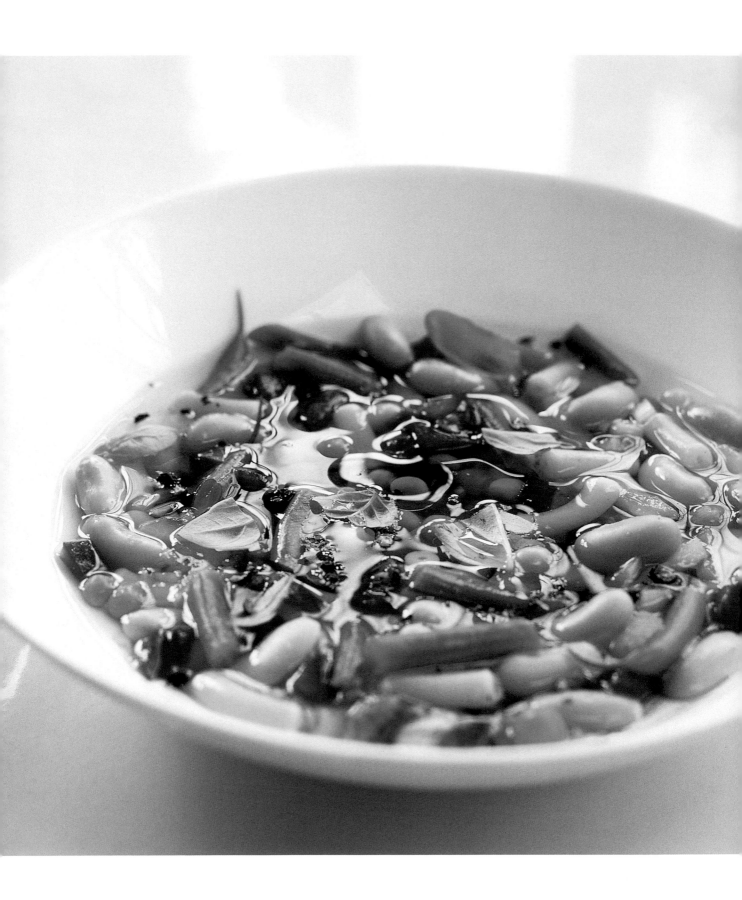

green macaroni minestrone

A twist on the classic minestrone, this fresh-tasting soup is full of vegetables, rich in fiber, and very satisfying—a real meal in itself. Enhanced with fresh tomatoes and basil, and drizzled with the finest olive oil, it is best served simply with good crusty bread.

SERVES 4

2/3 cup white wine
1 onion, peeled and minced
1 garlic clove, peeled and crushed
6 cups vegetable stock
2/3 cup macaroni
1 1/2 cups fine green beans, trimmed and cut into
 1-inch lengths
14 oz canned cannellini beans, drained and
 rinsed
1/2 cup frozen green peas
2 ripe tomatoes, chopped
3 tablespoons chopped basil
4 teaspoons extra virgin olive oil
freshly ground black pepper

1 Pour the white wine into a large pan and add the onion and garlic. Cover the pan and steam-fry for 6 minutes or until softened, stirring occasionally.

2 Add the stock and bring to a boil. Tip in the macaroni and cook for 6 minutes. Stir in the green beans and simmer for 3 more minutes, then add cannellini beans and peas, and simmer for a further 2 minutes.

3 Add the tomatoes and basil, and heat through for 1 minute. Season well with black pepper. Ladle the minestrone into four warm bowls and drizzle a teaspoon of extra virgin olive oil over each one.

veggie barley broth with garlic toasts

This hearty broth of root vegetables is full of fiber, which helps the body to absorb nutrients. It is thickened with pearl barley, which may sound rather old-fashioned, but barley is an excellent grain and very under-rated. It has a lovely, nutty flavor and a wonderful, almost creamy texture in soups and stews.

SERVES 4

6 cups chicken or vegetable stock

1/2 cup pearl barley

1 leek, trimmed

2 celery stalks

2 large carrots, peeled

1 medium parsnip, peeled

5 tablespoons white wine

2 tablespoons tomato paste

2 bay leaves

2 tablespoons chopped parsley

freshly ground black pepper

FOR THE GARLIC TOASTS:

1 rustic loaf, sliced

1 garlic clove, peeled and halved

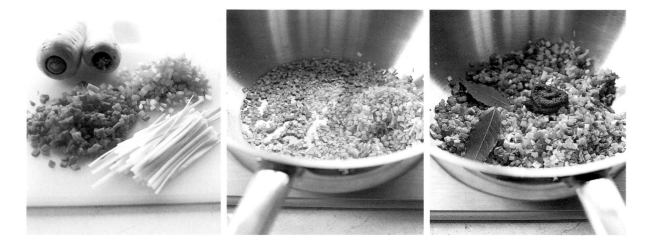

1 Pour the stock into a pan, add the pearl barley, and boil gently for 10 minutes. Meanwhile, mince the leek, celery, carrots, and parsnip.

2 Pour the wine into a large pan, add the leek, cover, and steam-fry for 5 minutes, stirring occasionally. Add the remaining vegetables and cook for a further 5 minutes.

3 Stir in the tomato paste, bay leaves, and pearl barley and stock mixture. Bring to a boil, then lower the heat and simmer for 15–20 minutes.

4 Meanwhile, toast the bread on both sides under the broiler, then rub with the garlic clove. Season the soup with pepper to taste and stir in the chopped parsley. Pour into warm bowls and serve, with the garlic toasts.

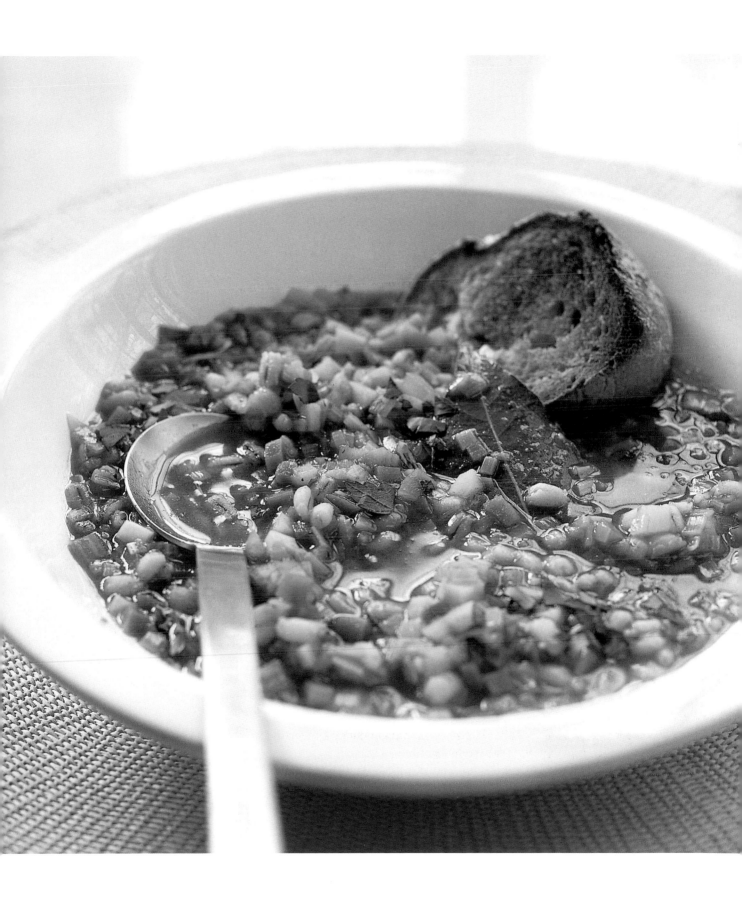

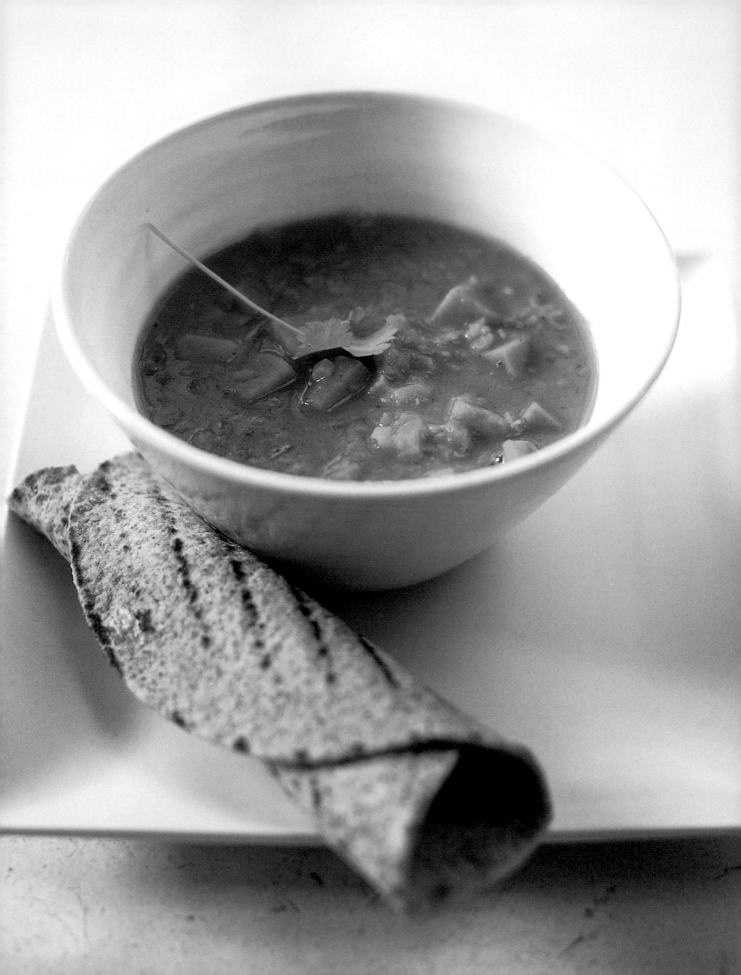

spiced red lentil and sweet potato soup

Quick-cooking red lentils and sweet potato cubes are spiced with medium or mild curry paste, then mellowed with coconut milk to make a comforting, warming soup. Lentils are full of fiber, which aids digestion, and they are a good source of vegetable protein. Serve this rich-textured soup with warm chapatti bread as a lunch or light supper.

SERVES 4

2 medium potatoes

1 large sweet potato

2 tablespoons curry paste, such as Madras or korma

1 onion, peeled and minced

²/₃ cup split red lentils

4 cups vegetable stock

1 cup coconut milk (preferably reduced-fat)

1–2 tablespoons chopped cilantro, plus sprigs for garnish

freshly ground black pepper

chapatti breads, for serving

1   Peel the potatoes and sweet potato, and cut into ½-inch cubes. Heat the curry paste in a pan, stir in the onion, cover, and steam-fry for 5 minutes, stirring occasionally.

2   Add the potatoes, sweet potato, lentils, and stock to the pan. Bring to a boil, then lower the heat and simmer for 20 minutes.

3   Stir in the coconut milk and gently heat through. Season to taste with pepper, then stir in the chopped cilantro. Ladle the soup into warm bowls, top with cilantro sprigs, and serve with warm chapatti breads.

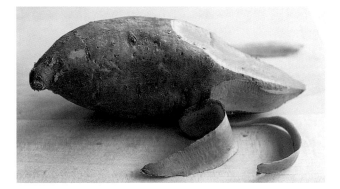

speedy soups

You can create tempting, flavorful soups without resorting to boiling up carcasses in the stockpot. Use aromatics like ginger, lemon grass, and chili peppers for an Asian-style pot, or try infusing water or light vegetable stock with sweet root vegetables, such as carrot, parsnip, and leek. Soups that are bursting with vegetables will only need water. For an instant, gently flavored stock, save your vegetable cooking water.

You can buy stocks or bouillon in cube or powdered form, or canned broths in cans. Seek out quality products, especially those that are salt-free. Stocks made from cubes and powders can be strong, so dilute with plenty of water. Toss in a few simple ingredients, such as chili pepper, noodles, and shrimp, or curry paste, chicken, and spinach, to transform your stock into a bowl of steaming goodness. Each of the following soups serves 4 as a first course or as a light meal with bread.

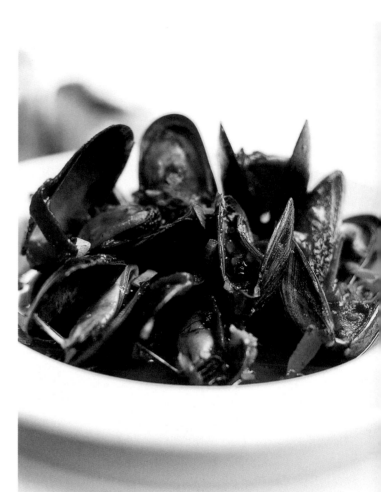

garlicky mussel bisque
Heat 1 tbsp olive oil in a large pan, stir in 3 crushed garlic cloves, and cook for 30 seconds. Add 2 lb scrubbed live mussels, 1½ cups arrabiatta sauce, and 1¼ cups red wine. Cover with a lid and cook for 2–3 minutes or until the mussels have opened; discard any that remain closed. Ladle into serving bowls, scatter chopped parsley over, and serve, with crusty, rustic bread.

curried chicken soup

Heat 2 tbsp curry paste in a pan and stir in 1 thinly sliced onion. Cover and cook for 5 minutes, stirring occasionally. Add 8 oz skinless chicken breast meat, cut into thin strips, and cook for 1 minute. Pour in 4 cups chicken stock, bring to a boil, and simmer for 5 minutes. Stir in 2 cups baby spinach leaves and 2 tbsp mango chutney. Heat through and season with pepper. Serve with warm chapatti bread.

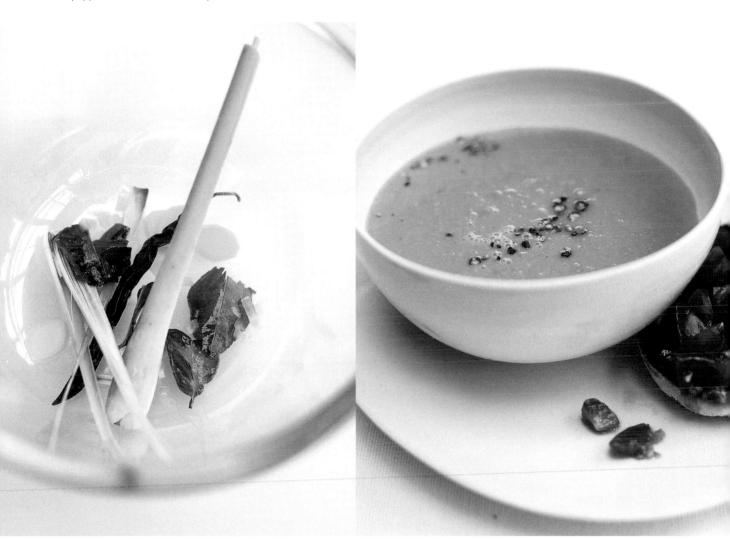

hot and sour soup

Heat 1 tsp peanut oil in a pan and stir in ½ tsp dried chili flakes, a 1-inch piece fresh ginger, peeled and minced, and 1 crushed garlic clove. Cook for 1 minute. Add 5 cups chicken stock and simmer gently for 10 minutes. Stir in 8 oz peeled, raw tiger shrimp, 1 tbsp Thai fish sauce, 1 cup halved sugarsnap peas, 4 oz rice noodles, and the grated zest and juice of 1 lime. Bring to a boil, then simmer for 3 minutes. Serve at once.

pea and basil soup with tomato bruschetta

Cook 1 chopped onion in 1 tsp olive oil in a covered pan for 8 minutes; stir occasionally. Add 4 cups vegetable stock and 3½ cups frozen green peas. Bring to a boil, then simmer for 3 minutes. Whiz in a blender until smooth, then reheat, stirring in 3 tbsp pesto sauce. Season with pepper. Serve with thick slices of toasted ciabatta (Italian slipper bread), rubbed with garlic and topped with chopped tomatoes and a drizzle of extra virgin olive oil.

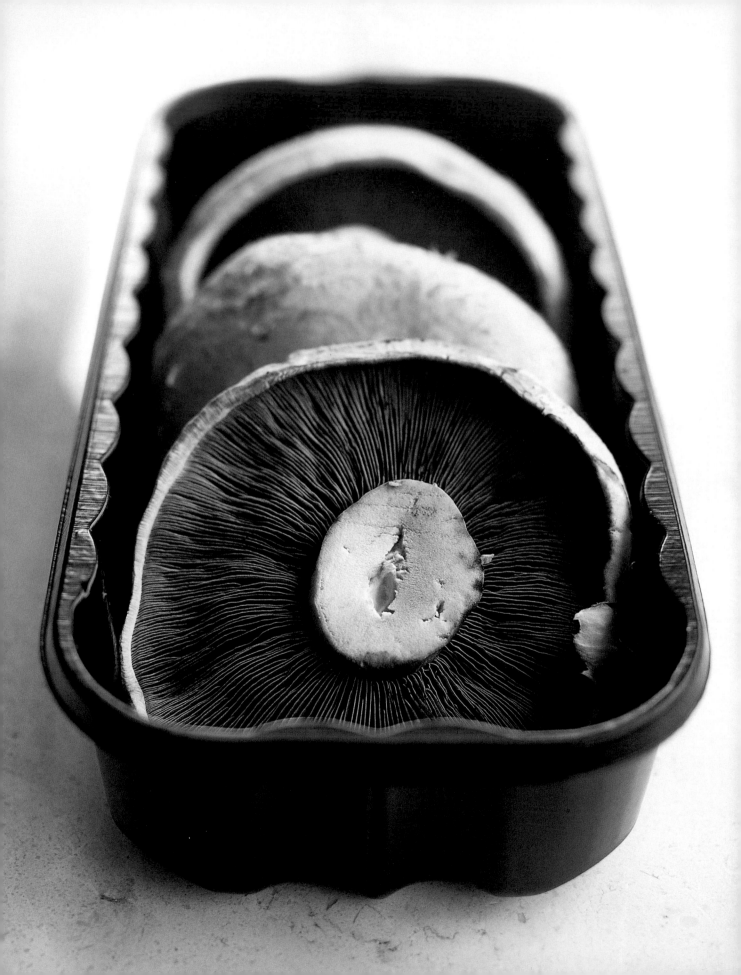

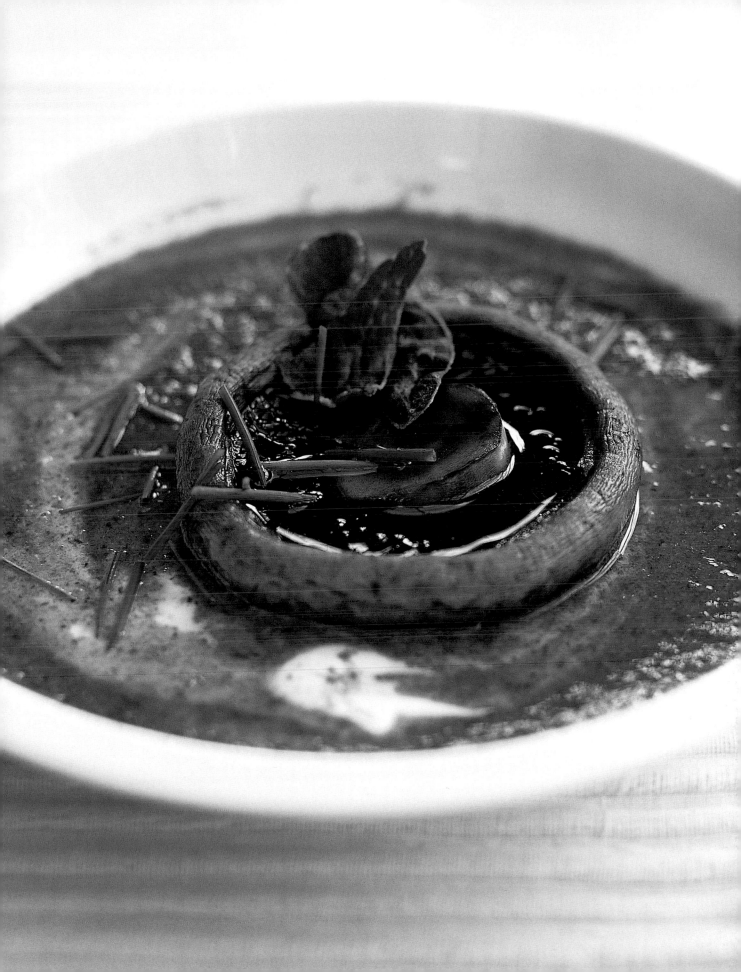

portobello mushroom and bacon soup

This wonderful, dark soup is intensely flavored with portobello mushrooms and thickened with a little whole-wheat bread. Mushrooms are rich in protein and also contain B vitamins and useful minerals. They are very low in calories, provided you fry them in the minimum of oil. The soup is finished with a tasty topping of broiled whole mushrooms and crisp prosciutto. *Illustrated on page 45*

SERVES 4

1¼ lb portobello mushrooms, plus 4 extra
   whole ones for serving
3 teaspoons olive oil
1 onion, peeled and minced
1 garlic clove, peeled and crushed
4 cups vegetable stock
2 small slices of whole-wheat bread, crusts
   removed
3 tablespoons crème fraîche or light sour cream
4 slices of prosciutto
1 tablespoon snipped chives
freshly ground black pepper

1   Peel and slice the mushrooms. Heat 2 teaspoons of the oil in a large pan. Add the onion and garlic, cover, and cook for 8 minutes or until soft, stirring occasionally.

2   Stir in the sliced mushrooms and cook for 4 minutes. Add the stock and bring to a boil. Lower the heat and simmer for 10 minutes. Add the bread to the pan and simmer for a further 5 minutes.

3   Pour the soup into a blender and whiz until smooth. Return to the pan, place over a low heat, and stir in the crème fraîche or sour cream. Season well with pepper.

4   Meanwhile, preheat the broiler. Place the 4 whole mushrooms, cup-side up, on a nonstick baking sheet. Drizzle the remaining olive oil over the mushrooms and grind some black pepper over. Broil for 3 minutes. Lay the prosciutto on the sheet alongside the mushrooms and broil for a further 1 minute or until the prosciutto is crisp.

5   Pour the hot soup into warm bowls and top each serving with a broiled mushroom, crisp prosciutto, and snipped chives.

Moorish shrimp and chick pea soup

Inspired by Middle Eastern flavors, this is a great pantry recipe that uses canned chick peas and tomatoes. Tomatoes contain lycopene, which is thought to help reduce the risk of certain cancers. Regular eating of fresh or processed tomatoes is said to lessen the risk of heart disease and bowel and prostate cancers. To serve, the soup is topped with fragrant couscous flavored with lemon, cilantro, and shrimp.

SERVES 4

$1/2$ cup couscous

2 cups tomato purée

14 oz canned crushed tomatoes with garlic

2 teaspoons harissa paste

$2/3$ cup white wine

14 oz canned chick peas (garbanzo beans),
  drained and rinsed

pinch of sugar

grated zest and juice of $1/2$ lemon

2 tablespoons extra virgin olive oil

5 oz cooked peeled shrimp

2 tablespoons chopped cilantro

freshly ground black pepper

1 Put the couscous into a bowl, pour $2/3$ cup boiling water over, and set aside to soak for 5 minutes until the water is absorbed.

2 Meanwhile, pour the tomato purée and crushed tomatoes into a pan and add the harissa paste and wine. Stir in the chick peas and heat gently for 5 minutes. Season to taste with black pepper and a pinch of sugar.

3 Fluff up the couscous with a fork. Add the lemon zest and juice, olive oil, shrimp, and cilantro, and toss to mix. Season with pepper to taste.

4 Pour the spicy tomato soup into four warm bowls, top with the couscous, and serve.

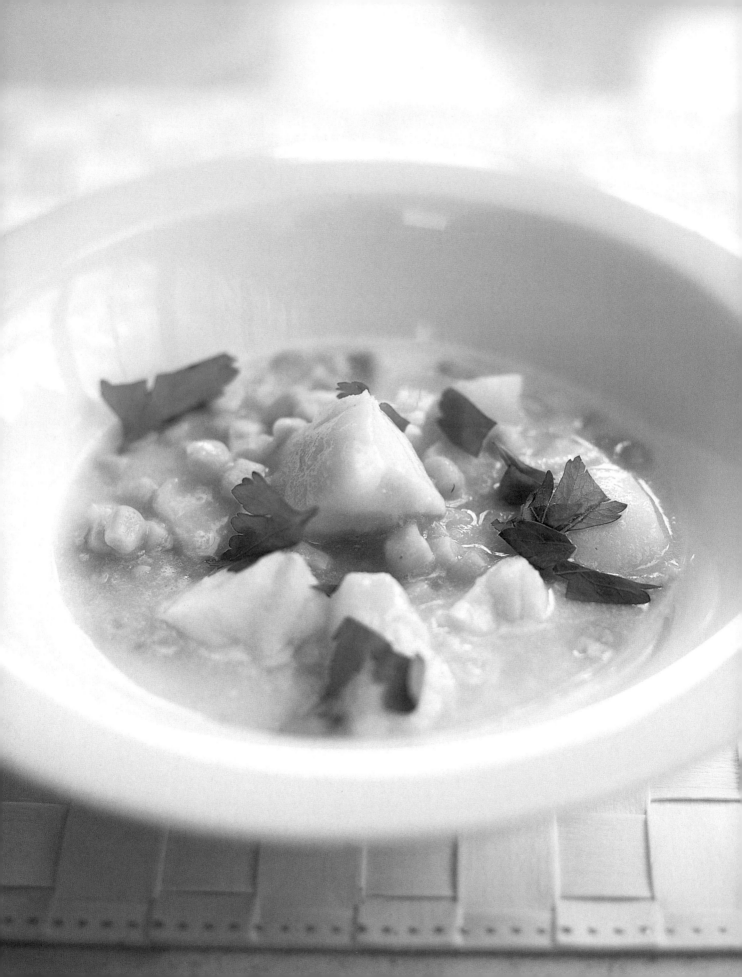

smoked fish chowder

This chunky soup is made with smoked fish, diced potatoes, and corn kernels. Smoked haddock and cod are packed with flavor and protein, yet they're very low in fat. Blitzing half the potatoes with the stock and milk gives the chowder a creamy texture without the addition of cream.

SERVES 4

2 teaspoons olive oil

1 onion, peeled and minced

3$^{1}/_{2}$ cups peeled and diced potatoes

2$^{1}/_{2}$ cups fish stock

1$^{1}/_{4}$ cups lowfat milk

1$^{1}/_{2}$ cups canned corn kernels in water, drained

1 lb skinless smoked haddock (finnan haddie) or
   smoked cod fillets, cut into bite-sized pieces

2 tablespoons chopped parsley

freshly ground black pepper

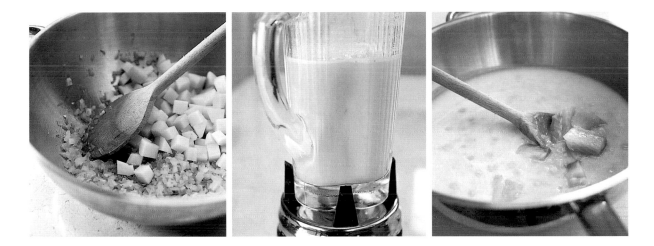

1 Heat the oil in a large pan, add the onion, and cook for 5 minutes. Add the diced potatoes and cook for 1 more minute. Pour in the stock and bring to a boil. Lower the heat, cover, and simmer for 12–15 minutes or until the potatoes are tender.

2 With a slotted spoon, remove half the potatoes from the stock and set aside. Pour the remaining soup into a blender, add the milk and whiz until smooth. Pour back into the pan.

3 Add the corn and simmer for 2 minutes. Stir in the fish pieces and reserved potatoes, and cook for a further 3–4 minutes. Stir in the chopped parsley and season with black pepper to taste. Ladle into four warm bowls and serve.

oodles of noodles soup

Rice noodles and chicken soak up all the fragrant Asian flavors in this simple broth. Miso is a traditional Japanese paste made from fermented soybeans. It is available in Japanese markets and wholefood stores. For the stock base, use 2–3 tbsp, or more to taste. Miso is rich in iron, while chicken is an excellent source of easily digested protein.

SERVES 4

5 cups miso broth
1 tablespoon grated fresh ginger
2 tablespoons good-quality soy sauce
8 oz skinless chicken breast meat, cut
  into thin strips
4 oz Thai stir-fry rice noodles
8 oz bok choy, divided into leaves
½ bunch green onions, chopped
2 teaspoons toasted sesame oil
freshly ground black pepper

1 Make up the miso broth according to the package directions. Pour into a large pan and add the ginger, soy sauce, and chicken strips. Bring to a boil and simmer for 3 minutes.

2 Add the rice noodles and bok choy and cook for a further 2 minutes. Stir in the green onions, and simmer for a final minute. Stir in the sesame oil, season with black pepper, and serve in warm bowls.

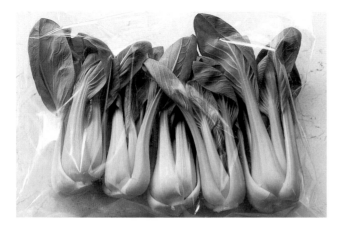

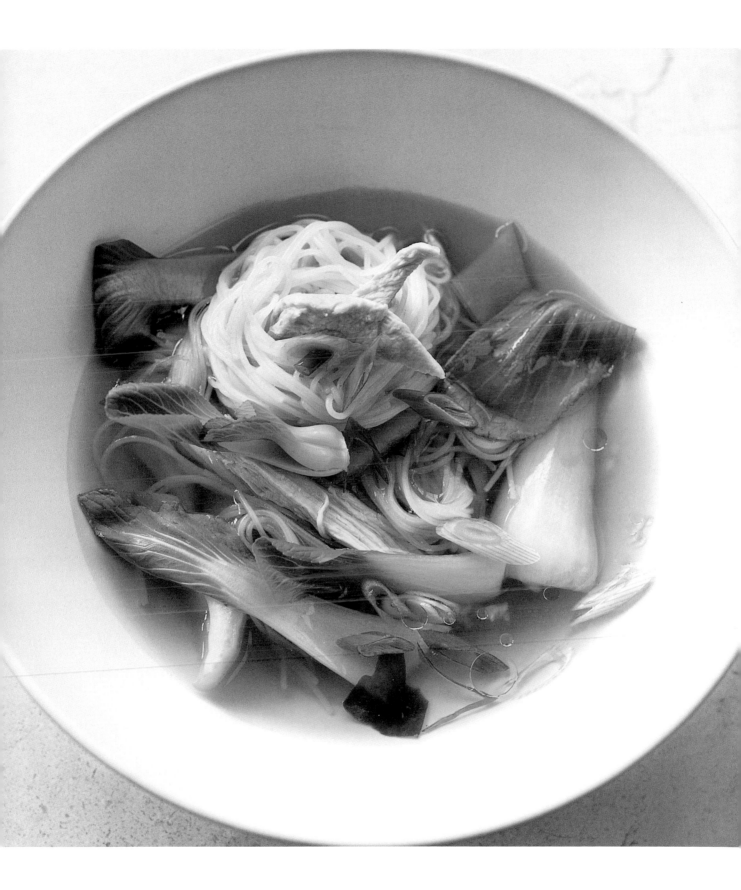

roasted zucchini and garlic soup

Roasting vegetables brings out their natural sweetness as they slowly brown in the oven and enhances the flavor of soups such as this. Zucchini are a good source of magnesium, which helps the body absorb other important minerals. Crème fraîche gives the soup a lovely creamy texture, while olive-flavored croûtons provide a crunchy contrast.

SERVES 4

2 lb zucchini
1 onion, peeled and cut into 8 wedges
3 garlic cloves (unpeeled)
1 tablespoon olive oil
5 cups vegetable stock
1 cup frozen green peas
1 black olive ciabatta (Italian slipper bread) or
  other rustic bread
3 tablespoons crème fraîche or light sour cream
freshly ground black pepper

1 Preheat the oven to 400°F. Thickly slice the zucchini into 1-inch chunks.

2 Place the zucchini, onion, and garlic in a roasting pan and toss with the olive oil. Season with pepper, then roast for 30–35 minutes or until golden and tender.

3 Pour the vegetable stock into a saucepan and bring to a boil. Add the peas and bring back to a boil, then lower the heat and simmer for 2 minutes until tender.

4 Remove the vegetables from the oven. Peel the garlic cloves. Transfer the roasted vegetables and garlic to a food processor or blender, add the stock and peas, and blend until smooth. (It may be necessary to purée the soup in batches.) Season with pepper to taste.

5 Cut the ciabatta into rough 1-inch cubes and place on a baking sheet. Toast in the oven for 5 minutes or until crisp. Meanwhile, pour the soup into the saucepan, stir in the crème fraîche or sour cream, and heat gently. Ladle the soup into warm bowls and serve with the croûtons.

gazpacho with lemon-feta bulgur wheat

This easy Mediterranean chilled soup is perfect for a summer lunch. Vitamin B-rich bulgur wheat has a good crunchy texture and it only needs to be soaked before use. Feta cheese, which is traditionally made from sheep's milk and cured in a salty brine, has a distinctive tang. It is a good source of calcium. Together the wheat and feta provide an original topping for the soup.

SERVES 4

14 oz canned crushed tomatoes
1¼ cups tomato juice
2 garlic cloves, peeled and crushed
1 tablespoon olive oil
2 tablespoons white wine vinegar
dash of Tabasco sauce
1 red bell pepper, halved, seeded, and diced
⅔ cup bulgur wheat
grated zest and juice of ½ lemon
3 oz feta cheese, crumbled
2 tablespoons chopped parsley
freshly ground black pepper

1 Place the tomatoes, tomato juice, garlic, olive oil, vinegar, and Tabasco in a food processor. Process until smooth. Season to taste with black pepper and stir in the red bell pepper. Chill the soup for at least 15 minutes.

2 Tip the bulgur wheat into a bowl, pour ½ cup boiling water over, and set aside to soak for 10 minutes. Fork through the bulgur wheat, then stir in the lemon zest and juice, feta, and parsley. Season to taste.

3 Ladle the chilled soup into individual bowls. Just before serving, top each portion with a spoonful of the lemon and feta bulgur wheat.

3 fish

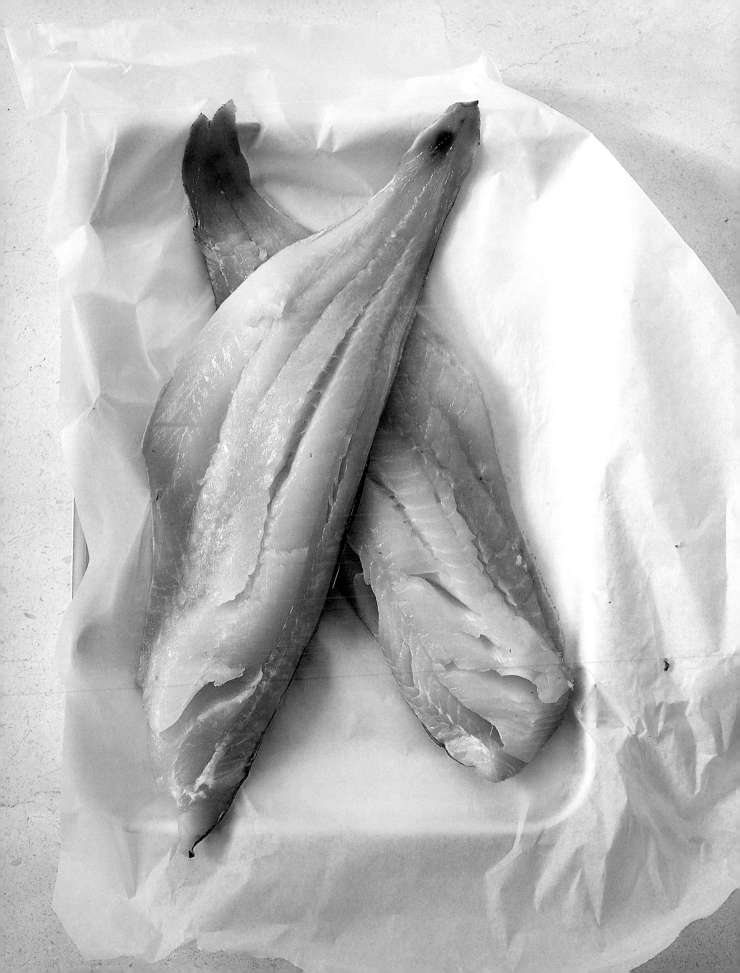

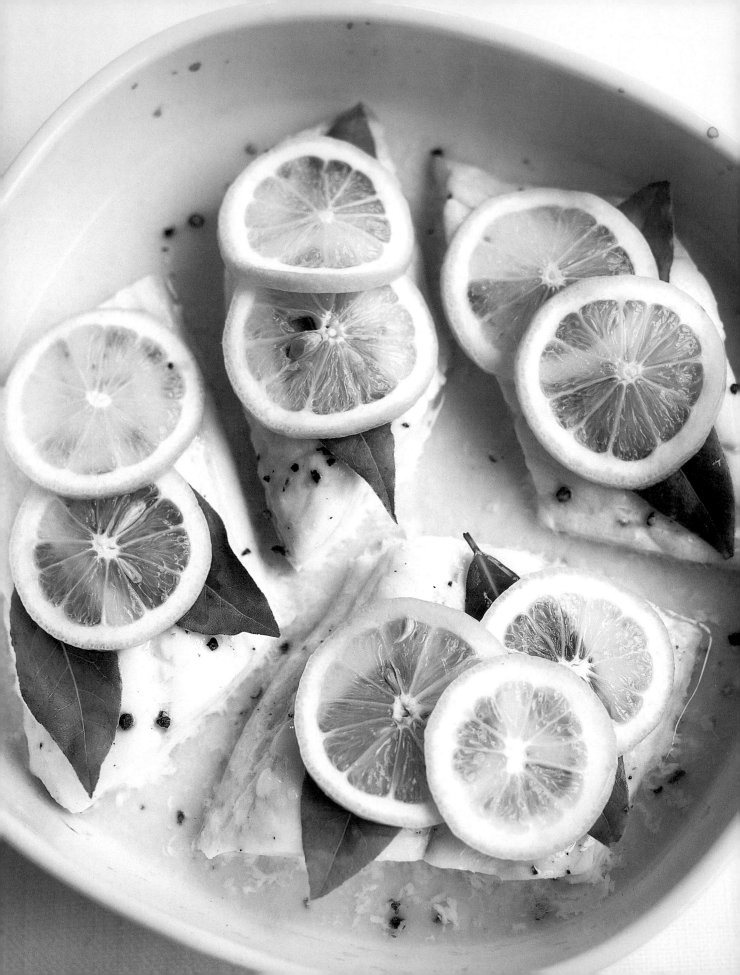

lemon and bay-scented hoki with piquant mash

Hoki is a firm white fish from New Zealand, similar to haddock and cod, which can also be used in this recipe. Here, it is simply baked with aromatic bay and some dry vermouth (you could also use white wine or even fish stock). With the fish serve a creamy and tasty mash, made without butter and cream, but with mustard and plain yogurt.

SERVES 4

4 skinless hoki or haddock fillets, each about
  5 oz
8 bay leaves
1 lemon, thinly sliced
4 tablespoons dry vermouth
freshly ground black pepper
FOR THE MASH:
2 lb potatoes, peeled
4 tablespoons plain yogurt
3 tablespoons warm milk
2 tablespoons grain mustard

1   Preheat the oven to 375°F. For the mash, cut the potatoes into equal-sized chunks and place in a pan of cold water. Bring to a boil, then lower the heat and simmer for 20 minutes or until tender.

2   Meanwhile, arrange the fish fillets in a baking dish and season with black pepper. Place 2 bay leaves on each fish fillet and cover with slices of lemon. Drizzle with the vermouth and cover with damp parchment paper. Bake for 10–12 minutes or until the fish is just opaque.

3   Drain the potatoes well and tip back into the pan. Mash over a gentle heat until smooth. Stir in the yogurt, milk, and mustard, then season to taste.

4   Serve the hoki with the mustard-flavored mash, and sugarsnap peas or snow peas.

mustard-crusted cod with bell peppers and beans

Cod steaks keep wonderfully moist underneath an unusual crisp topping of couscous, which is soaked in cold rather than hot water for extra crunch. Red bell peppers and green beans provide color and plenty of vitamin C.

SERVES 4

6 tablespoons couscous

2 tablespoons Dijon mustard

4 cod steaks, each about 5 oz

3 red bell peppers

1 tablespoon olive oil

12 oz green beans, trimmed and sliced

squeeze of lemon juice

freshly ground black pepper

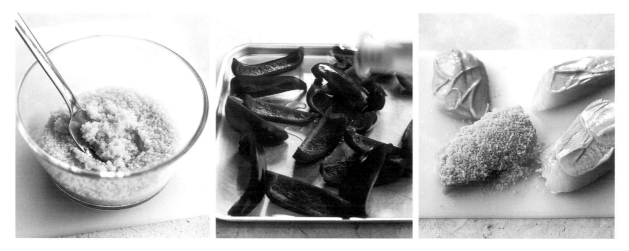

1 Preheat the oven to 400°F. Place the couscous in a small bowl, pour ½ cup cold water over, and let soak for 5 minutes.

2 Spread the mustard evenly over the cod steaks, sprinkle the couscous on top, and press to adhere. Set to one side.

3 Halve, core, and seed the peppers, then cut each half into 4 strips. Place the pepper strips in a roasting pan, drizzle the olive oil over, and toss well to coat with the oil. Roast for 25–30 minutes.

4 Toss the green beans in with the peppers and season with black pepper. Set the cod steaks on top, couscous side up, and squeeze the lemon juice over them. Roast for 8–10 minutes. Serve hot.

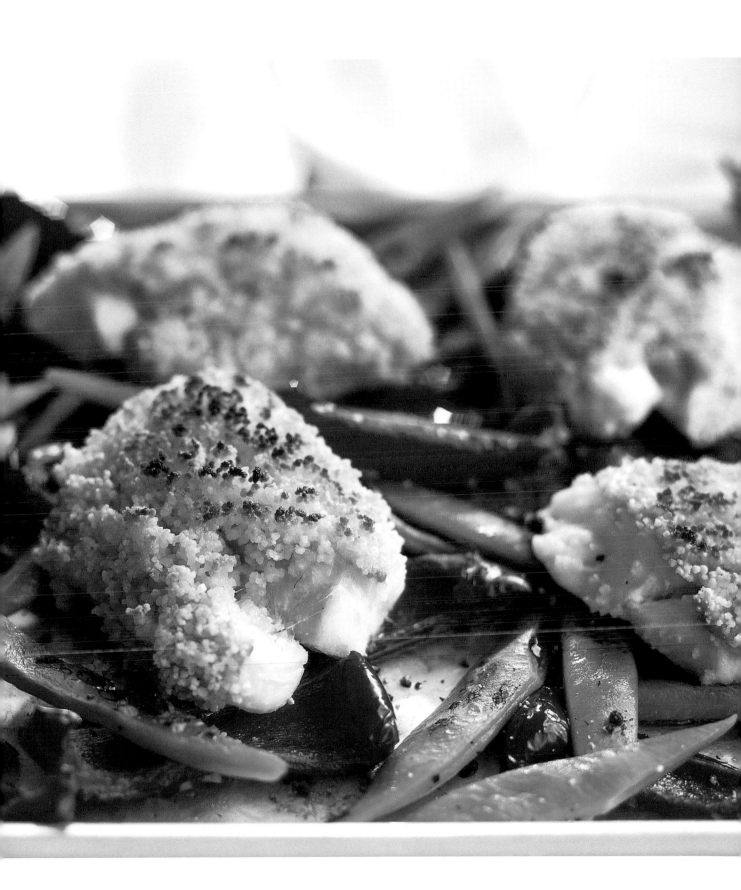

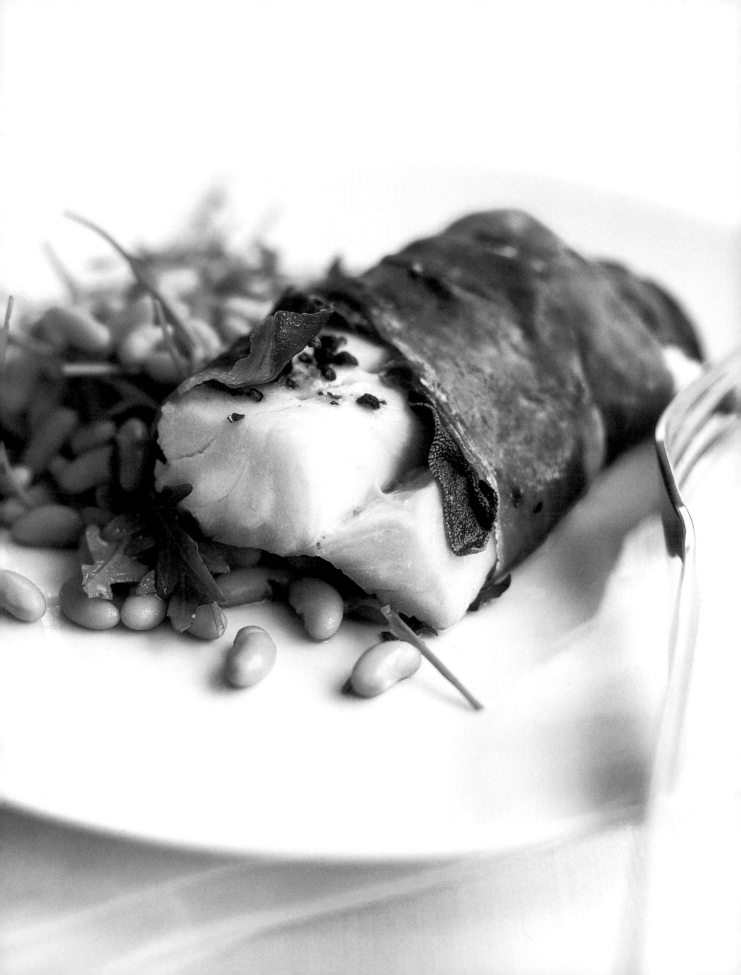

prosciutto-roasted cod with bean and arugula salad

I find that prosciutto and meaty fish work well together, as their flavors really complement each other. Garlic and lemon enhance the flavor of flageolet beans, and fresh arugula provides a delicious, peppery contrast.

SERVES 4

4 skinless pieces of cod fillet, each about 5 oz
12 sage leaves
4 slices of prosciutto
14 oz canned flageolet beans, drained and
  rinsed
2 garlic cloves, peeled and crushed
2 tablespoons extra virgin olive oil
1 tablespoon lemon juice
2 handfuls arugula leaves
freshly ground black pepper

1   Preheat the oven to 425°F. Season the cod with black pepper. Arrange 3 sage leaves on each cod fillet and wrap in a slice of prosciutto. Place in a roasting pan and roast for 6–8 minutes, depending on the thickness of the cod.

2   In the meantime, tip the flageolet beans into a pan. Add the garlic and stir over a medium heat for 2 minutes or until heated through. Add the olive oil and lemon juice, and season well. Add the arugula leaves and stir through the beans.

3   Divide the bean and arugula salad among four serving plates and place a portion of roasted prosciutto-wrapped cod alongside. Serve hot.

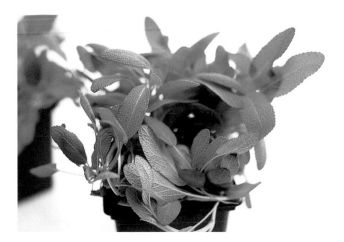

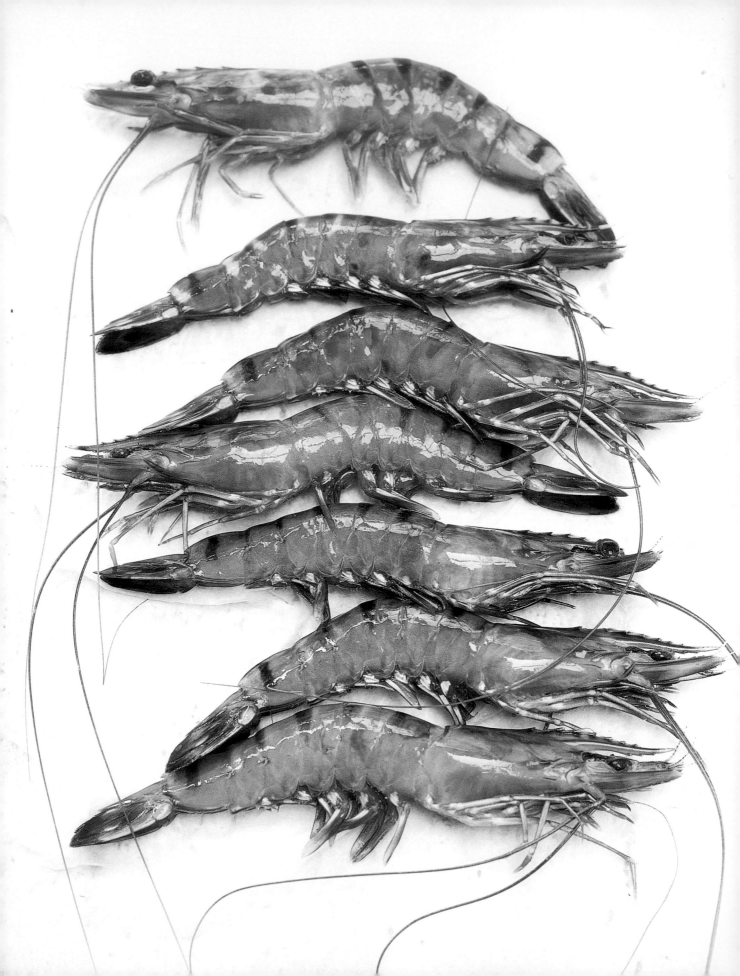

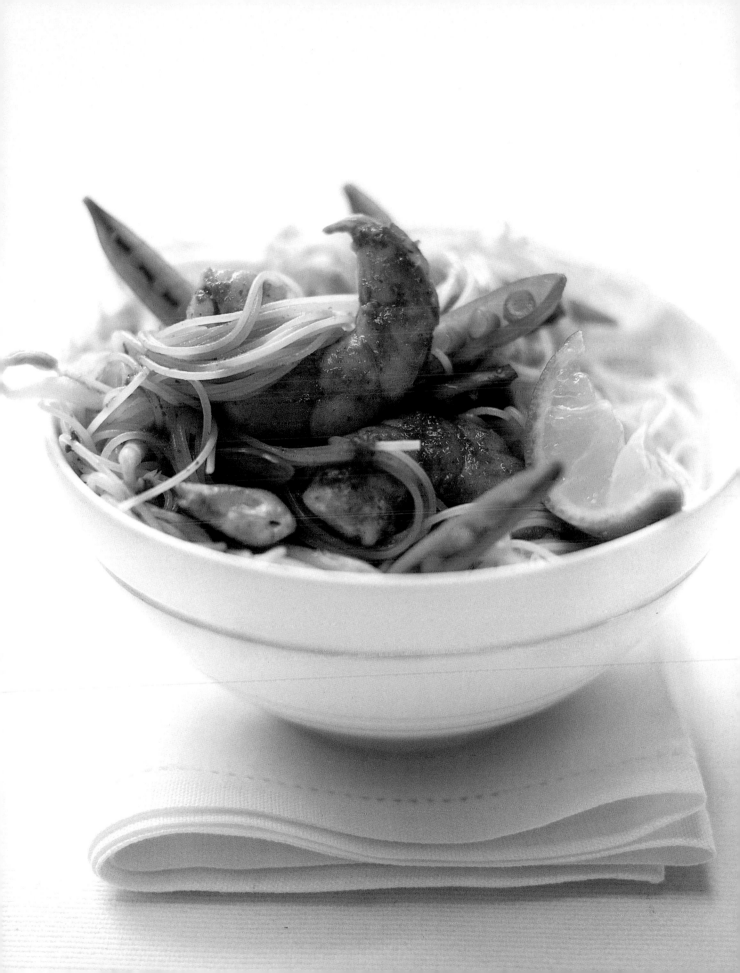

tiger shrimp and red Thai noodles

Rice noodles are a lighter alternative to the more familiar Chinese egg noodles. Here, they are combined with juicy tiger shrimp and crunchy vegetables for a tempting stir-fry that can be made in less time than it takes to pick up the phone and order a takeout. Instead of tiger shrimp, you can use any raw jumbo or very large shrimp. To prepare the shrimp, simply twist off the head and tail, peel away the shell from the body, and remove the dark intestinal vein. *Illustrated on page 63*

SERVES 4

1½ tablespoons Thai red curry paste

4 tablespoons tomato purée

4 oz Thai rice noodles

8 oz raw tiger shrimp, peeled and deveined

1½ cups sugarsnap peas, halved lengthwise

1½ cups bean sprouts

⅓ cup cashew nuts, toasted

lime wedges for serving

1 Mix the Thai red curry paste and tomato purée together in a small bowl and set aside. Cook the rice noodles according to the package directions, then drain.

2 Meanwhile, heat a nonstick wok until very hot, add the shrimp, and cook for 1 minute. Add half the red Thai paste mix and stir-fry for a further minute. Add the sugarsnap peas along with 2 tablespoons water and stir-fry for 2 minutes.

3 Stir in the rice noodles, bean sprouts, cashew nuts, and remaining red Thai paste mix. Toss over a high heat for a further 2 minutes until piping hot. Divide the shrimp noodles among four warm bowls and serve immediately, with lime wedges.

teriyaki swordfish with spinach and coconut

This tasty dish presents a real infusion of flavors. A teriyaki marinade adds an Asian touch to firm, meaty swordfish, while the accompanying coconut gravy—based on coconut milk—is full of aromatic spices. The pan-grilled swordfish is served on a bed of leaf spinach, a good source of iron, calcium, and vitamins A and C.

SERVES 4

4 swordfish steaks, each about 5 oz
2 teaspoons olive oil
4 tablespoons teriyaki sauce
1 garlic clove, peeled and crushed
2 tablespoons Madras curry paste
1 tablespoon tomato paste
14 oz canned coconut milk (preferably
  reduced-fat)
squeeze of lemon juice
12 oz baby spinach leaves (about 3¹/₂ cups)
freshly ground black pepper

1   Place the swordfish steaks in a non-metallic dish and season with pepper. Mix together the olive oil, teriyaki sauce, and garlic, then drizzle this over the swordfish. Set aside for 5 minutes.

2   Heat a medium saucepan, add the curry paste and tomato paste, and fry for 30 seconds. Pour in the coconut milk and simmer for 5 minutes. Finish with a squeeze of lemon juice to taste.

3   Heat a nonstick grill pan until very hot. Add the swordfish steaks and pan-grill for 2–3 minutes on each side. Pour in the teriyaki marinade and bubble, spooning it over the swordfish steaks to glaze.

4   In the meantime, put the spinach in a large pan (with just the water clinging to the leaves after washing), cover, and cook for 30 seconds or until just wilted. Stir and season with a little pepper.

5   Place the wilted spinach in the center of each serving plate, top with the swordfish steaks, and drizzle the coconut gravy over.

smoked haddock tortilla

This Spanish-style omelet, packed full of smoked haddock, potatoes, and onions, is easy to make and a rich source of protein. You could also make it with smoked whitefish or smoked cod. Cooking the onions slowly brings out their natural sweetness, which complements the spicy fava bean and tomato salsa.

SERVES 4–6

1 lb medium waxy potatoes, peeled and
  halved
8 oz skinless smoked haddock (finnan haddie)
  fillet
2 teaspoons olive oil
2 large, mild onions, peeled and finely sliced
6 eggs
freshly ground black pepper
FOR THE SALSA:
2 cups baby fava or lima beans, cooked and
  skinned
3 plum tomatoes, chopped
1 tablespoon tomato ketchup
large dash of Tabasco sauce

1 Parboil the potatoes in water for 8–10 minutes until only just tender, then drain. When cool enough to handle, thickly slice the potatoes. Cut the smoked haddock into thin slivers and set aside.

2 Heat the olive oil in a large nonstick frying pan (suitable for use under the broiler). Add the onions, cover, and steam-fry for 5 minutes, stirring occasionally. Remove the lid and cook for 8 minutes or until the onions are soft and golden. Stir in the sliced potatoes and cook for a further 2 minutes.

3 Preheat the broiler. Beat the eggs in a bowl and season with pepper. Pour the beaten eggs into the frying pan and scatter the smoked haddock slivers on top. Cook the tortilla, gently shaking the pan, for 4 minutes or until it is just set on the base.

4 Place the pan under the broiler and cook the tortilla for a further 3 minutes or until golden and just set on top. Meanwhile, mix the salsa ingredients together in a bowl and season with pepper to taste.

5 Turn the tortilla onto a warm serving plate and cut into wedges. Serve immediately, with the tomato and fava bean salsa.

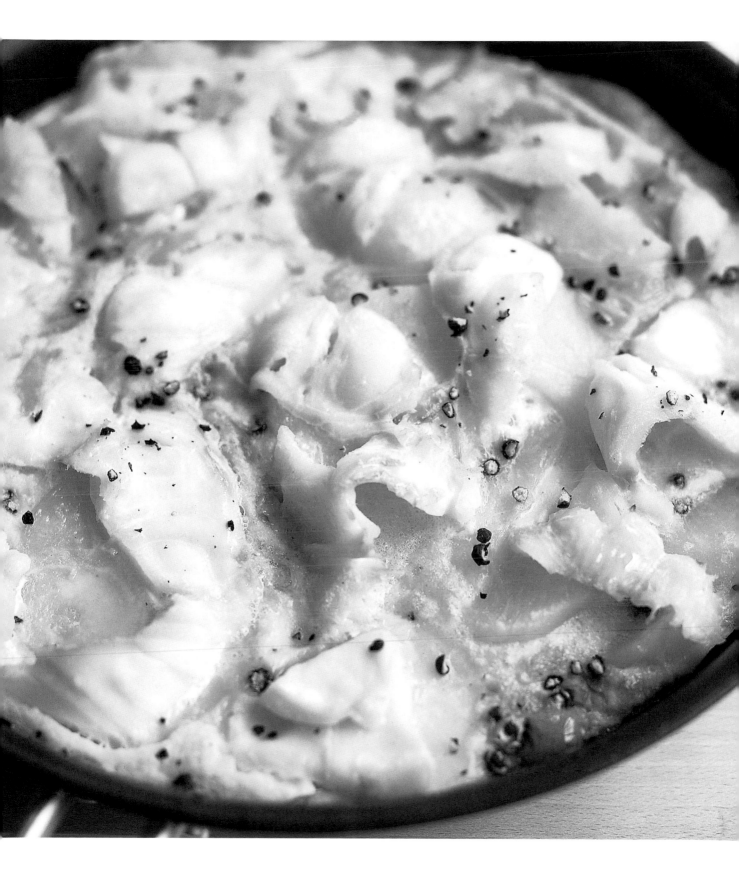

seared tuna with green beans and basil

Fresh tuna is rich in healthy fish oils, the omega-3s. These oils are beneficial because they help to maintain a healthy heart. Blanching the green beans for just a few minutes in boiling water before plunging them into cold water helps to retain their color and nutrients.

SERVES 4

1 teaspoon olive oil

4 fresh tuna steaks, each about 5 oz

2 tablespoons balsamic vinegar

1 lb baby new potatoes

8 oz fine green beans, trimmed

8 oz cherry tomatoes, halved

1/2 bunch of green onions, trimmed and minced

freshly ground black pepper

FOR THE PISTOU:

2 garlic cloves, peeled

large bunch of basil

2 tablespoons extra virgin olive oil

juice of 1/2 orange

1   Sprinkle the olive oil over the tuna steaks and rub in with your fingertips. Place in a non-metallic dish, grind some pepper over, and drizzle the balsamic vinegar over the fish. Set aside for 15 minutes.

2   Boil the potatoes until tender, then drain and set aside to cool. Add the green beans to a pan of boiling water and blanch for 2–3 minutes, then drain and refresh in cold water. Drain thoroughly, then tip into a bowl. Add the potatoes, tomatoes, and green onions, and toss to mix.

3   To make the pistou, put the garlic, basil, olive oil, and orange juice into a small food processor and process until blended. Season to taste.

4   Heat a nonstick grill pan until it is really hot. Add the tuna steaks and pan-grill for approximately 2 minutes on each side until cooked.

5   Pour two-thirds of the pistou over the salad and gently mix together. Arrange the salad on four serving plates, top each with a tuna steak, and spoon the remaining pistou on top. Serve at once.

pan-fried smoked salmon salad with avocado

For a different way of serving smoked salmon, try it quickly flashed in a hot pan and served with salad, avocado, and a warm tomato and chive dressing. Avocado is rich in vitamin E, a good source of potassium, and high in monosaturated fatty acids.

SERVES 4

2 plum tomatoes
3 tablespoons olive oil
1 bunch of chives, roughly chopped
juice of 1/2 lemon
8 oz smoked salmon slices
4 oz mixed salad leaves
1 large, ripe avocado, halved, pitted, peeled,
  and sliced
freshly ground black pepper

1 Immerse the plum tomatoes in a bowl of boiling water for 30 seconds or so, then remove and peel away the skin. Halve, seed, and thinly slice the tomatoes.

2 Heat 2 1/2 tablespoons olive oil in a small pan. Add the plum tomatoes, chives, and a large squeeze of lemon juice. Season to taste and gently heat through.

3 Heat the remaining olive oil in a nonstick frying pan. Add the salmon pieces, grind a little black pepper over, and cook for 30 seconds on each side.

4 Divide the salad leaves among four serving plates and top with the avocado slices. Arrange the smoked salmon slices, slightly folded, on the avocado. Spoon the hot tomato and chive dressing over the top, and serve at once.

oily fish

Oily fish is a great source of protein and rich in the beneficial omega-3 oils. It is tasty, readily available, and moderately priced, and we should all aim to eat some once or twice a week.

Buy fresh oily fish on the day you are going to eat it. If the fish are whole, check that they have clear eyes and gleaming skin. Fillets and steaks should look and smell fresh. However you cook your fish, don't overdo it, or it will become dry.

Of course, you don't have to buy fresh to enjoy oily fish, because it is the original convenience food. Simply reach to your cupboard for a nutritious can of salmon, mackerel, anchovies, or sardines. These fabulous little cans can be transformed into the quickest of suppers—squashed onto bread, popped into a hot baked potato, and even blitzed with cream cheese for an instant pâté to serve with crusty bread. Each of the following recipes serves 4.

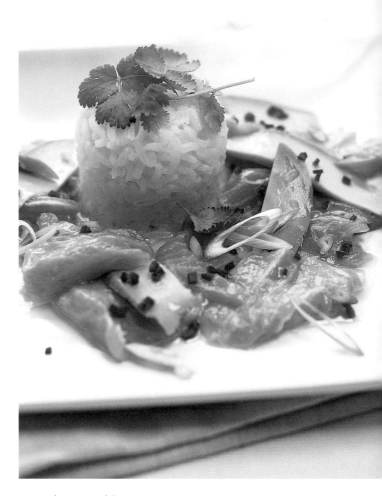

salmon sushi

Thinly slice 1 lb skinless salmon fillet crosswise; lay in a dish. Mix 2 tbsp extra virgin olive oil, juices of 1 lemon and 1/2 lime, 1 minced hot red chili pepper, and 4 finely sliced green onions. Scatter onto the salmon and marinate for 20 minutes. Cook 1 cup Thai fragrant rice; cool slightly, then toss with juice of 1/2 lime and pepper to taste. Pack into cups, unmold onto plates, and top with cilantro. Surround with the salmon and thin avocado slices. Spoon the marinade over to serve.

anchovy and tuna potatoes

Rub 4 scrubbed baking potatoes all over with 1 tsp olive oil and bake at 400°F for about 1 hour until tender. Drain 14 oz canned white-meat tuna in water and 14 oz canned cannellini beans. Toss together, along with 2 oz canned anchovy fillets, minced with their oil, 1 finely sliced red onion, grated zest and juice of 1 lemon, 4 tbsp chopped parsley, and pepper. Split the baked potatoes and fill with the tuna salad.

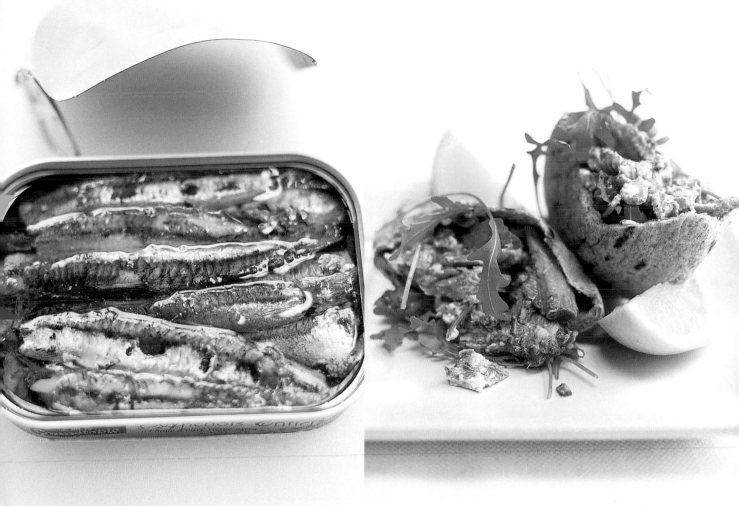

baked oaty mackerel fillets

Lay 8 mackerel fillets, flesh-side up, on a nonstick baking sheet. Spread with 4 tbsp grain mustard and coat with 10 crushed small oat crackers. Bake at 400°F for 10 minutes. Meanwhile, peel and chop 4 tart apples and cook in a pan with the grated zest and juice of ½ lemon for 5–6 minutes until tender but still holding shape. Stir in 2 tsp thyme leaves and pepper to taste. Serve the mackerel with the apple sauce and green beans or another green vegetable.

lemon and sardine pitas

Mix ½ cup cream cheese with the grated zest of 1 lemon and pepper to taste. Gently stir in 8 oz canned sardines in tomato sauce, keeping the mixture chunky. Brush 4 whole-wheat pita breads with a little olive oil and cook in a hot nonstick grill pan for 1 minute each side until charred and crisp. Split the pita breads open and divide the sardine mixture among them. Top each with a handful of arugula leaves and serve with lemon wedges.

seared trout with sweet potato wedges

Trout is an oily fish that is high in protein and contains those helpful omega-3 oils. I cut the sweet potatoes into chunky pieces so they don't absorb too much oil, and leave the skins on, to keep the wedges in shape and provide added fiber. You can use white potatoes if you prefer—they'll just take a little longer to cook. A piquant citrus and caper dressing complements the richness of the trout beautifully.

SERVES 4

3 medium sweet potatoes, scrubbed
2 tablespoons Worcestershire sauce
3 tablespoons olive oil
2 large rainbow trout, filleted

juice of 1 large orange
juice of 1/2 lemon
2 tablespoons small capers, drained
1 tablespoon chopped parsley
freshly ground black pepper

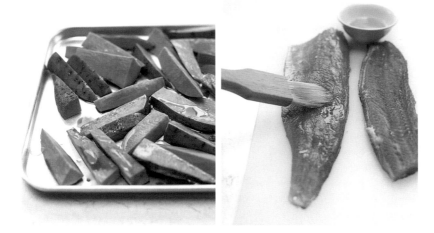

1 Preheat the oven to 400°F. Cut the sweet potatoes into thick wedges and place in a large bowl. Add the Worcestershire sauce and 2 tablespoons olive oil, and toss to mix. Transfer to a large roasting pan and season with pepper. Bake for 30–35 minutes until golden and crisp.

2 Meanwhile, heat a nonstick grill pan until very hot. Brush the flesh side of the trout fillets with the remaining olive oil and season well with pepper. Place the fillets, flesh-side down, in the grill pan and cook for 2 minutes each side. Remove from the pan and arrange on serving plates.

3 Add the orange and lemon juices, capers, and parsley to the grill pan and bubble for a few seconds. Spoon the warm dressing over the trout fillets and serve, with the roasted sweet potato wedges.

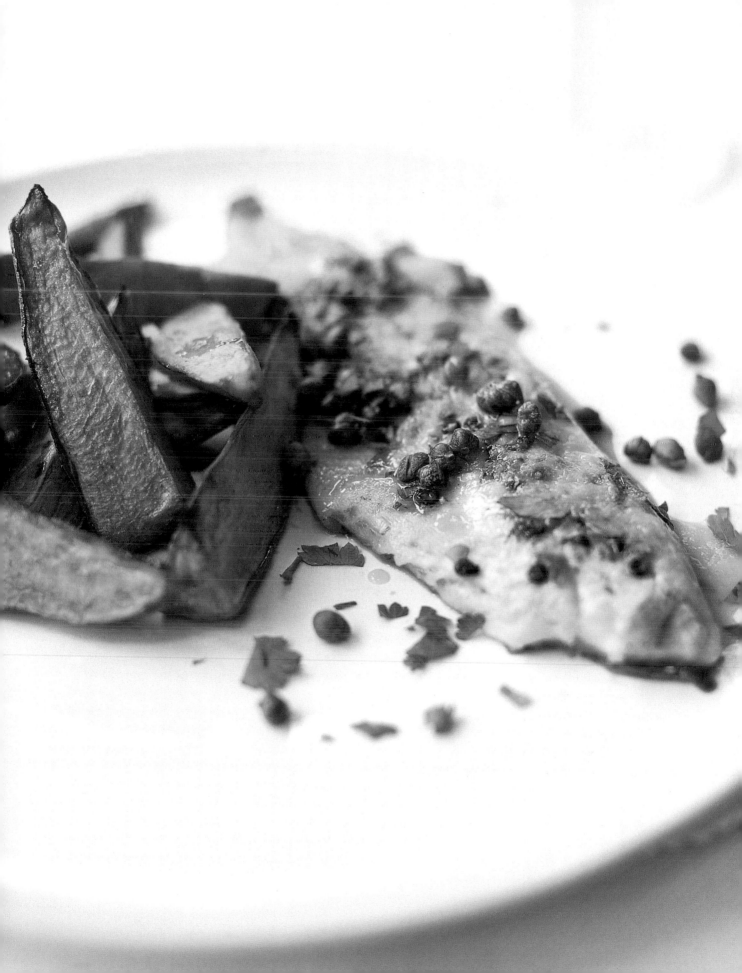

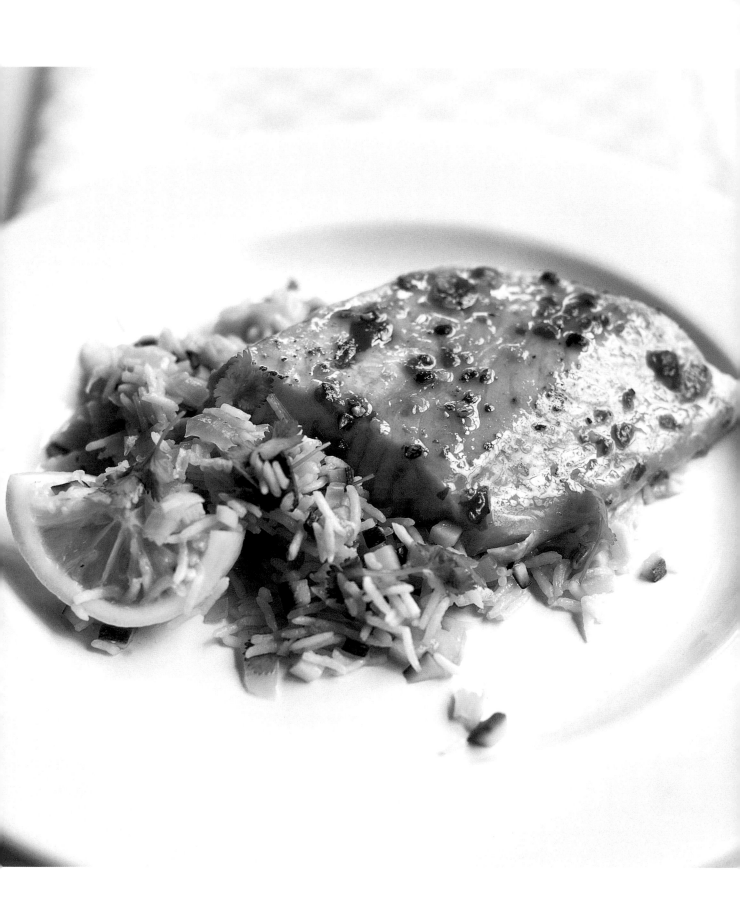

chili salmon with zucchini and lemon pilaf

Just a touch of chili brings out all the fresh flavors in this dish, which is packed with protein and vitamins. As the lemon is added unpeeled to the pilaf, be sure to scrub it well with hot soapy water and then rinse before use.

SERVES 4

1¹/₃ cups basmati rice

2 teaspoons olive oil

1 onion, peeled and minced

2 garlic cloves, peeled and crushed

4 zucchini, chopped

1 small lemon, cut into quarters

2¹/₂ cups vegetable stock

4 skinless pieces of salmon fillet, each about 5 oz

4 teaspoons sweet chili dipping sauce

3 tablespoons chopped cilantro

freshly ground black pepper

1 Rinse the basmati rice in a strainer under cold running water, then set aside to drain.

2 Heat the olive oil in a large, shallow pan. Add the onion and garlic, and cook gently for 5 minutes or until softened. Stir in the rice, zucchini, and lemon quarters, and cook for 1 minute.

3 Pour in the stock and bring to a boil. Cover and cook over a low heat for 15 minutes until all the stock has been absorbed and the rice is tender.

4 Meanwhile, preheat the broiler. Lay the salmon on a nonstick baking sheet, grind some black pepper over, and spread each fillet with a teaspoon of chili sauce. Broil for 5–6 minutes or until cooked through and lightly charred.

5 Season the pilaf to taste and stir in the chopped cilantro. Spoon onto four serving plates, discarding the lemon if you prefer, and place the salmon fillets alongside.

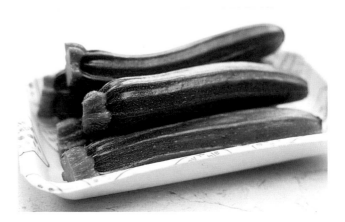

roasted salmon on black toasts

Steam, pan-grill, or bake rather than deep-fry fish, to create flavorful dishes using the minimum of fat. Here, baked salmon strips are served on tangy olive tapenade toasts—a lowfat alternative to a hollandaise or other creamy sauce. Top with a zesty, peppery salad that provides iron and vitamin C for a healthy lunch or supper.

SERVES 4

1¼-*lb piece thick salmon fillet*
juice of ½ lemon
1 tablespoon olive oil
4 thick slices of ciabatta (Italian slipper bread)
4 tablespoons black olive tapenade
FOR THE SALAD:
1 bunch of watercress, trimmed
1 red onion, peeled and thinly sliced
2 large oranges, segmented
freshly ground black pepper

1 Preheat the oven to 400°F. Cut the salmon into 8 equal strips and lay these on a nonstick baking sheet. Drizzle the lemon juice and half the olive oil over the fish, and season with pepper. Bake for 8–10 minutes or until the salmon is just cooked.

2 For the salad, toss the watercress sprigs, onion slices, and orange segments together in a bowl. Season with a little pepper.

3 Meanwhile, heat a large nonstick grill pan and brush with the remaining oil. Pan-grill the ciabatta slices for 2 minutes each side or until golden and crisp. Spread the ciabatta toasts with the olive tapenade and place on four serving plates. Lay two strips of salmon on each toast. Top with the salad and serve.

spiced mackerel with spinach lentils

The spinach lentils in this healthy dish can easily be made ahead if required and then reheated. Lentils are extremely nutritious, being a good source of protein, fiber, vitamin B, calcium, iron, and phosphorus. Here, they are served with spiced mackerel—a fine fish that's rich in beneficial omega-3 oils.

SERVES 4

2 tablespoons coriander seeds
1 tablespoon coarsely ground black pepper
4 tablespoons roughly chopped Italian parsley
8 small mackerel fillets
1 tablespoon olive oil
FOR THE SPINACH LENTILS:
1 tablespoon sunflower oil
1 large onion, peeled and chopped
4 garlic cloves, peeled and crushed
1 tablespoon garam masala
2 cups split red lentils, rinsed
5 cups vegetable stock
4 cups roughly chopped spinach leaves

1 To release the flavor from the coriander seeds, pound with a mortar and pestle, or place them in a plastic bag and crush with a rolling pin. Tip into a bowl and mix with the pepper and parsley.

2 Rub the flesh side of the mackerel fillets with olive oil, then sprinkle with the spice mix and press to adhere. Set to one side.

3 For the spinach lentils, heat the sunflower oil in a large pan. Add the onion and steam-fry for 5 minutes. Add the garlic and garam masala and cook for a further minute. Stir in the lentils and stock, bring to a boil, and simmer for 15–20 minutes or until the lentils are just tender.

4 Heat a nonstick grill pan over a medium heat. When hot, add the mackerel fillets, skin-side down, and cook for 2–3 minutes. Turn carefully and cook for a further 2 minutes.

5 Stir the spinach into the lentils and cook briefly until just wilted. Spoon onto four serving plates and top each serving with two mackerel fillets.

4 chicken and turkey

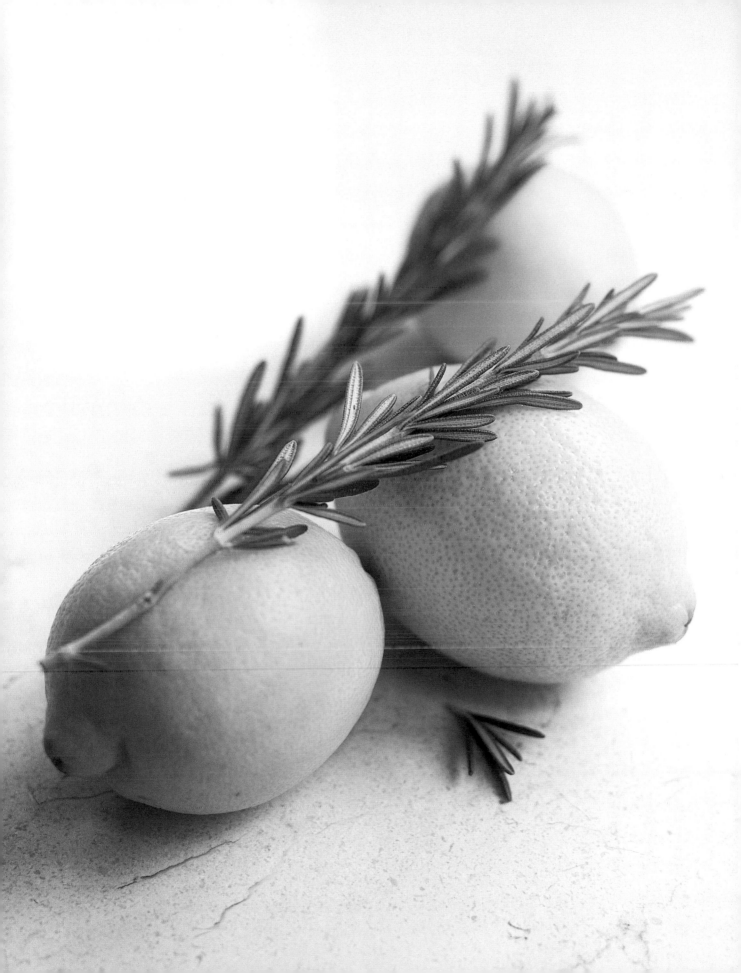

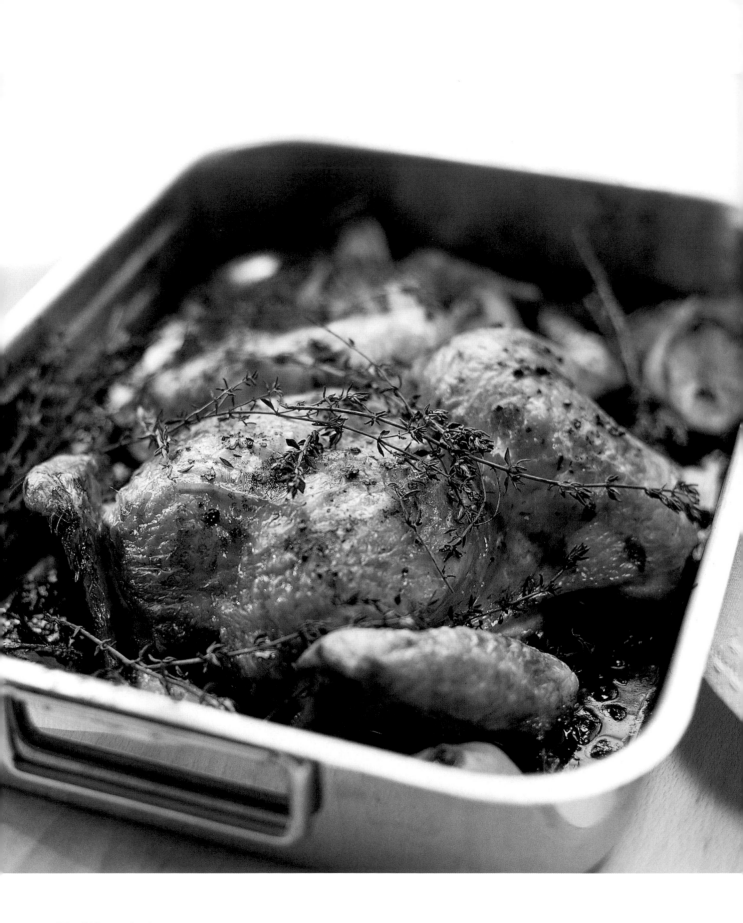

citrus-roasted chicken with tzatziki

This is one of my favorite ways of cooking chicken. Removing the backbone and flattening the bird helps it to cook more quickly and evenly, keeping the breast meat moist. I like to serve this citrus roast with a homemade tzatziki, but if time is short you can use a bought version.

SERVES 4

1 free-range or organic chicken, about 3¹/₂ lb
handful of thyme sprigs
1 large orange, cut into quarters
2 lemons, halved
freshly ground black pepper
FOR THE TZATZIKI:
¹/₂ hothouse cucumber
1 cup thick plain yogurt
1 garlic clove, peeled and crushed
1 tablespoon extra virgin olive oil
¹/₂ cup chopped mint leaves
lemon juice, to taste

1   Preheat the oven to 400°F. Lay the chicken, breast-side down, on a board. Using poultry shears, cut down either side of the backbone. Turn the chicken over and press to flatten, using the heel of your hand. Season generously with pepper and place, breast-side down, in a roasting pan. Scatter the thyme over, then roast for 30 minutes.

2   Remove the roasting pan from the oven and reduce the setting to 350°F. Squeeze the juice from the orange and lemons over the chicken, then add the squeezed citrus pieces to the pan and turn the chicken over. Roast for a further 30–40 minutes until the chicken is cooked through. To test, use an instant-read thermometer: it should register 170°F in the thigh and 160°F in the breast.

3   Meanwhile, make the tzatziki. Coarsely grate the cucumber and squeeze out excess liquid, then place in a bowl. Add the yogurt, garlic, olive oil, mint, and lemon juice and black pepper to taste.

4   Remove the chicken from the oven, cover with foil, and let rest in a warm place for 10 minutes before carving. Serve the chicken with the tzatziki and a watercress salad.

cornmeal-crusted chicken

These crisp-baked chicken thighs, coated in Cajun-spiced cornmeal, are equally delicious hot or cold. Cornmeal is a good source of carbohydrate and it is gluten-free, so is especially useful for anyone with an intolerance to this wheat-based protein.

SERVES 4

8 skinless, boneless chicken thighs
juice of 1 lime
2 tablespoons Cajun spice mix
4 tablespoons cornmeal
1/2 tablespoon olive oil
1 large onion, peeled and sliced

3 red bell peppers, cored, seeded, and sliced
pinch of sugar
1 large garlic clove, peeled and crushed
2/3 cup vegetable stock
2/3 cup tomato juice
freshly ground black pepper
watercress sprigs for serving

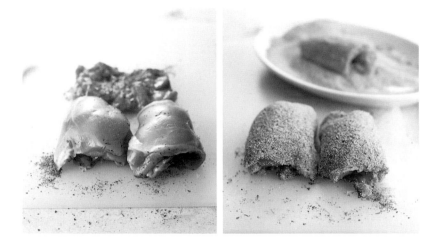

1 Preheat the oven to 400°F. Open out the chicken thighs and squeeze the lime juice over. Sprinkle with half of the Cajun spice, then shape into neat rolls.

2 Toss the cornmeal with the remaining Cajun spice and spread out on a plate. Turn the rolled chicken thighs in the cornmeal to coat evenly, pressing with your fingertips to ensure the coating adheres. Transfer the chicken to a roasting pan and bake for 35–40 minutes until golden and cooked through.

3 Meanwhile, heat the oil in a large pan. Add the onion and bell peppers, cover with a damp piece of parchment paper, and put the lid on the pan. Cook gently for 15 minutes until very soft. Stir in the sugar, garlic, stock, and tomato juice. Cover again and cook for a further 10 minutes. Cool slightly, then whiz in a blender or food processor until smooth. Season with pepper to taste.

4 Serve the cornmeal-crusted chicken with the red pepper gravy and watercress sprigs. Roasted new potatoes (see page 86) make an excellent accompaniment.

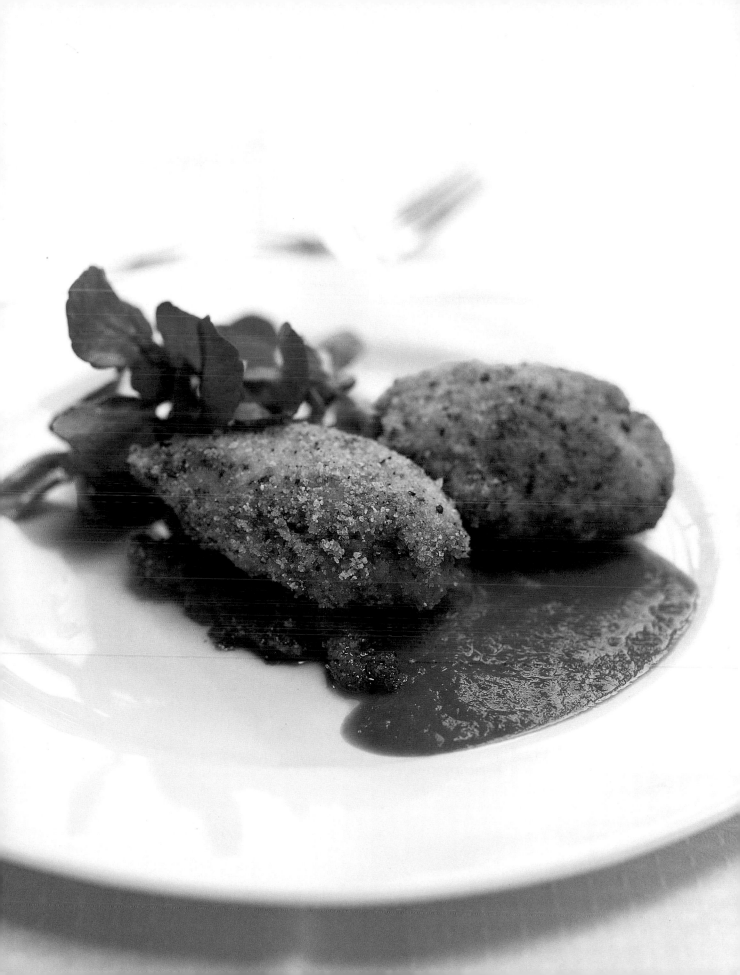

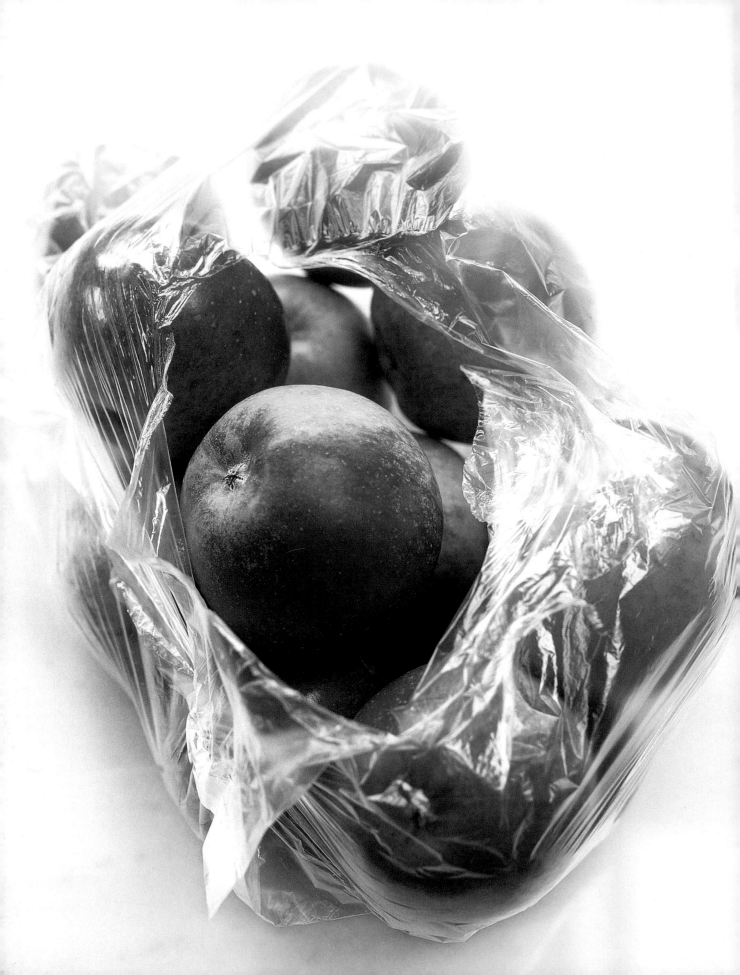

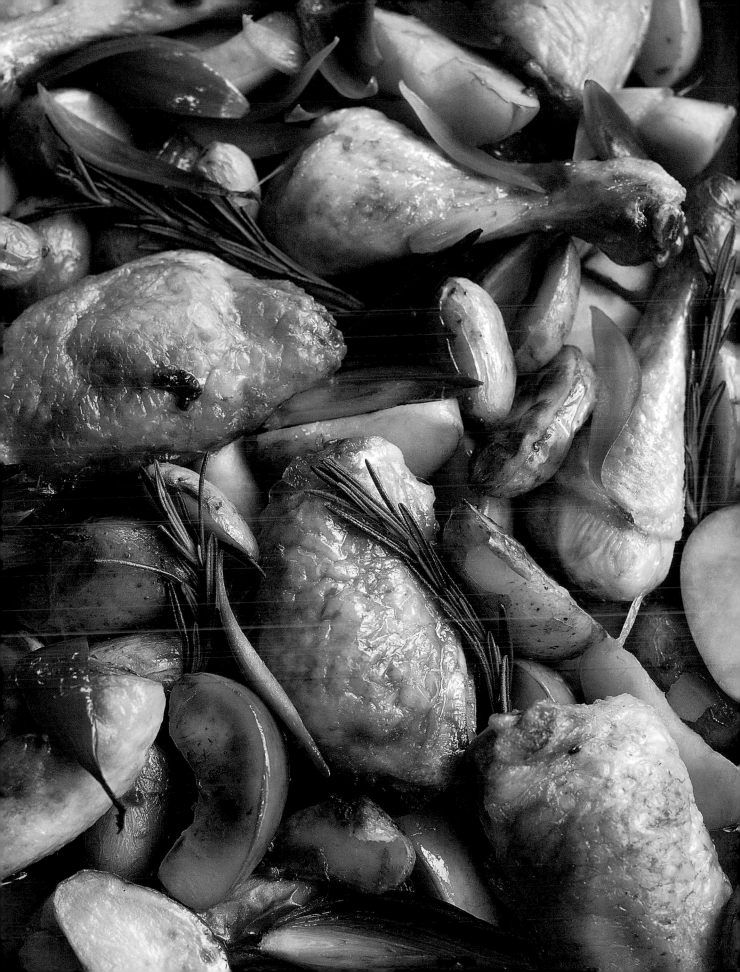

apple-roast chicken and new potatoes

Roasting chicken on the bone keeps it moist and tasty. To crisp the skin and lose as much fat as possible, the chicken pieces here are first roasted on a rack, then on a bed of apples flavored with rosemary and hard cider. Apples provide vitamin C and fiber. *Illustrated on page 85*

SERVES 4

4 free-range or organic chicken thighs

4 free-range or organic chicken drumsticks

juice of 1/2 lemon

1 tablespoon olive oil

2 red onions, peeled, halved, and each half cut into 4 chunks

1 cup hard cider

2/3 cup chicken stock

3 tart apples, cored and each cut into 6 wedges

3 rosemary sprigs

FOR THE ROASTED NEW POTATOES:

1 1/2 lb new potatoes, halved lengthwise

2 teaspoons olive oil

1 Preheat the oven to 400°F. For the roasted potatoes, place the potatoes in a roasting pan and drizzle the 2 teaspoons olive oil over them. Roast in the top of the oven for 35–40 minutes until tender and crisp.

2 Place the chicken, skin-side up, on a rack set in a roasting pan and squeeze the lemon juice over. Roast on a shelf below the potatoes for 20–25 minutes.

3 Meanwhile, heat the oil in a pan and steam-fry the onions over a medium heat for 10–15 minutes until beginning to soften and brown. Remove the paper or lid and pour in the cider and stock. Bring to a boil and simmer gently for 5 minutes.

4 Transfer the chicken pieces to a plate. Remove any fat from the roasting pan, then pour in the onion and cider. Add the apples and rosemary, then set the chicken pieces, skin-side up, on top. Roast for a further 15–20 minutes until the chicken is cooked through. Serve with the roasted potatoes.

maple-roasted squab chickens

Squab chickens make a change from a larger bird. You could also use Rock Cornish game hens. Here the birds are flavored simply with rosemary and garlic, and glazed with maple syrup to delicious effect. I like to serve them with hot new potatoes and a curly endive and walnut salad.

SERVES 4

4 squab chickens
4 rosemary sprigs
4 garlic cloves, peeled and lightly crushed
2 tablespoons maple syrup
1 tablespoon Dijon mustard
2 teaspoons olive oil
freshly ground black pepper

1 Preheat the oven to 400°F. Stuff the chicken cavities with the rosemary and garlic, then loosely tie up the legs with kitchen string.

2 In a small bowl, mix together the maple syrup, mustard, olive oil, and some black pepper. Place the chickens in a roasting pan and pour the maple syrup glaze over them.

3 Roast for 40–45 minutes, basting occasionally, until golden and cooked through. Serve with hot new potatoes and a crisp salad or green vegetable.

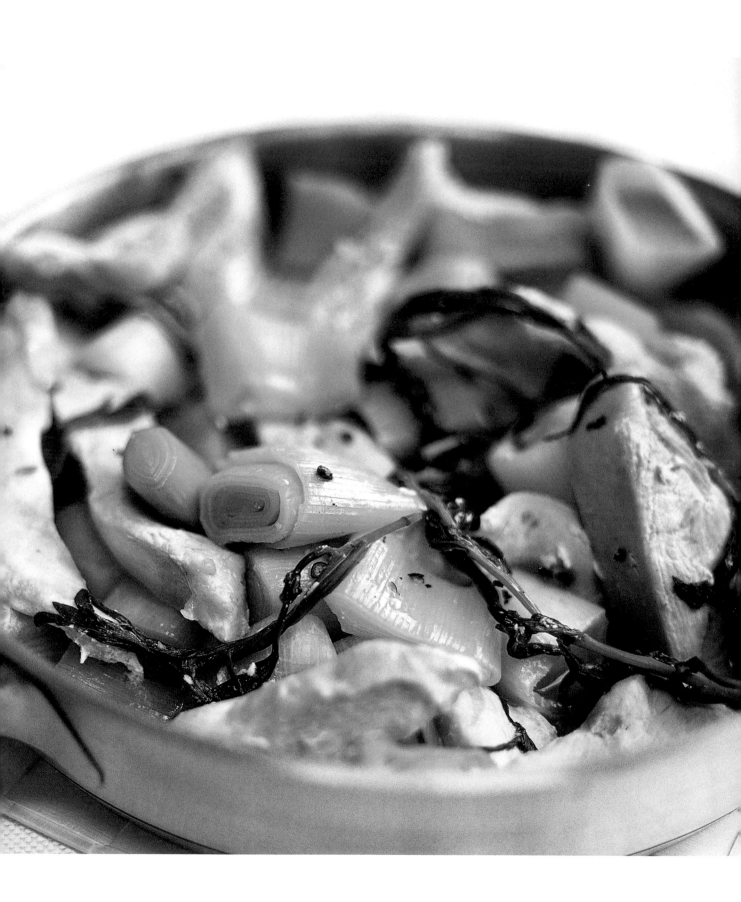

88 chicken and turkey

steamed tarragon chicken

Gently steaming chicken breasts with leeks and aromatic tarragon is a healthy way of cooking and keeps the meat succulent and full of flavor. A creamy, lowfat mustard and tarragon sauce is the perfect partner. All you need is a simple accompaniment, such as baked potatoes.

SERVES 4

4 boneless, skinless chicken breast halves, each about 5 oz
4 leeks, trimmed
1 tablespoon olive oil
2/3 cup white wine
8 tarragon sprigs
freshly ground black pepper

FOR THE SAUCE:

5 tablespoons crème fraîche or light sour cream
1 garlic clove, peeled and crushed
2 teaspoons Dijon mustard
2 tablespoons chopped tarragon

1 Cut each of the chicken breast halves lengthwise into 4 pieces. Slice the leeks into 3/4-inch pieces. Heat the olive oil in a large sauté pan, add the leeks, and gently steam-fry for 10 minutes. Add the wine and boil rapidly until it has almost totally reduced.

2 Scatter the tarragon sprigs over the leeks and lay the chicken pieces on top. Season with black pepper. Cover with a damp piece of parchment paper and put the lid on the pan. Cook very gently for 15–18 minutes until the chicken is cooked.

3 Meanwhile, to make the sauce, combine the crème fraîche or sour cream, garlic, mustard, and chopped tarragon in a bowl and stir until evenly blended. Season with pepper to taste.

4 Serve the steamed chicken and leeks with the creamy tarragon sauce.

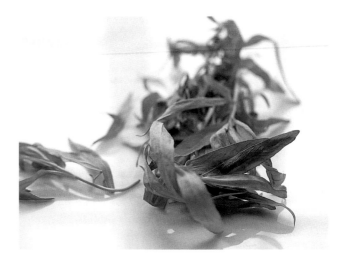

tomato-stuffed chicken pockets

Chicken breast halves are filled with sun-dried tomatoes and cream cheese, then wrapped in Italian pancetta and baked. A healthy stir-fry of Italian-style greens flavored with garlic, a hint of olive oil, and a squeeze of lemon is the perfect complement.

SERVES 4

4 boneless, skinless chicken breast halves, each
* about 5 oz*
4 tablespoons lowfat cream cheese
12 sun-dried tomatoes, drained and chopped
4 slices of pancetta or bacon
freshly ground black pepper

FOR THE GREENS:

1 tablespoon olive oil
2 garlic cloves, peeled and crushed
3 cups finely shredded cavolo nero or other
* hearty greens*
squeeze of lemon juice

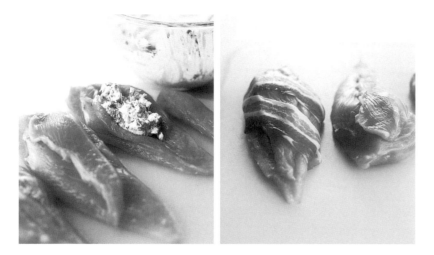

1 Preheat the oven to 400°F. Remove the small fillet from the underside of each chicken breast half and set aside. Make a vertical cut down the length of each chicken breast, but not all the way through, to form a pocket.

2 Mix the cream cheese with the tomatoes and season with pepper. Put a spoonful into each chicken breast pocket. Fold over the flaps of the pocket and cover with the reserved fillets to enclose the filling.

3 Loosely wrap a slice of pancetta around each chicken breast. Heat a stovetop-to-oven casserole, add the chicken, and sear for 2 minutes on each side until golden. Transfer to the oven and bake for 12–15 minutes or until the chicken is cooked through. (If you don't have a stovetop-to-oven casserole, start with a nonstick frying pan and then transfer the chicken to a roasting pan.)

4 Just before serving, heat the olive oil in a nonstick wok, add the garlic, and fry gently for 30 seconds. Add the shredded greens and stir-fry for 3–4 minutes until wilted, but still retaining a bite. Add a squeeze of lemon juice and pepper to taste. Serve the chicken breasts on the stir-fried greens.

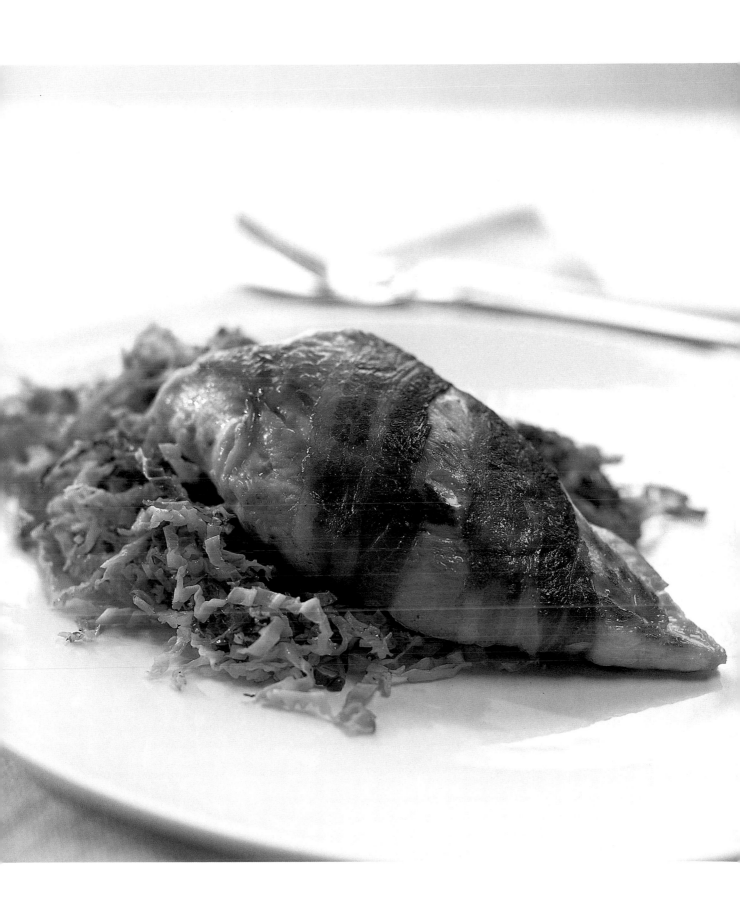

tapenade chicken with lemon lentils

Tapenade, or black olive paste, is one of the jewels in my pantry. It has so many uses, including making a tasty stuffing for chicken. I wrap these stuffed chicken breasts in prosciutto and serve them on lemony lentils—another pantry favorite. Lentils don't need to be soaked before cooking, and they're a good source of B vitamins, iron, and fiber.

SERVES 4

4 boneless, skinless chicken breast halves, each
   about 5 oz
4 tablespoons black olive tapenade
4 slices of prosciutto
4 bay leaves
1 teaspoon olive oil
freshly ground black pepper
FOR THE LEMON LENTILS:
1 1/2 cups lentils
4 cups chicken or vegetable stock
4 tablespoons extra virgin olive oil
grated zest and juice of 1 lemon
2 1/2 cups baby spinach leaves

1 Preheat the oven to 400°F. Put the lentils in a pan and pour in the stock. Bring to a boil and simmer for 20–25 minutes until the lentils are tender.

2 Meanwhile, place the chicken breast halves on a board and remove the small fillet from the underside of each breast; set aside. Make a vertical cut down the length of the chicken breast, but not all the way through, to create a pocket. Season all over with pepper.

3 Place a tablespoon of olive tapenade in the pocket of each chicken breast. Fold over the flaps of the pocket and cover with the reserved fillets to enclose the filling. Wrap a piece of prosciutto around each chicken breast and tuck in a bay leaf. Brush lightly with the olive oil.

4 Heat a stovetop-to-oven casserole, add the chicken, and sear for 2 minutes on each side until golden. Transfer to the oven and bake for 12–15 minutes or until the chicken is cooked through. (If you don't have a stovetop-to-oven casserole, start with a nonstick frying pan and then transfer the chicken to a roasting pan.)

5 When cooked, drain the lentils and return to the pan. Stir in the olive oil and lemon zest and juice. Return to the heat and gently warm through, then add the spinach and stir until wilted. Season with pepper to taste. Serve the chicken with the lentils.

chicken and prune ragout

I am a huge fan of juicy prunes, keeping a supply in my cupboard for healthy instant snacking. Prunes are rich in fiber and antioxidants, and they go well in savory dishes. Don't be put off by the number of garlic cloves in this recipe—they mellow and sweeten as they roast in their skins. Serve this ragout with couscous, rice, or fluffy mashed potatoes.

SERVES 4

3 large red onions, peeled and each cut into
   8 wedges
2 tablespoons olive oil
8 garlic cloves (unpeeled)
4 boneless, skinless chicken breast halves, each
   about 5 oz
1 cup red wine
1$^1/_2$ cups prunes
4 thyme sprigs
$^2/_3$ cup hot chicken stock

1   Preheat the oven to 400°F. Put the onion wedges in a roasting pan and drizzle 1 tablespoon olive oil over them. Roast for 20 minutes, then add the garlic cloves and roast for a further 10 minutes.

2   Meanwhile, using a small knife, slash the top of each chicken breast half in a criss-cross fashion, taking care not to cut all the way through. Put the chicken pieces in a shallow dish and pour the remaining olive oil and ¼ cup of the red wine over them. Let marinate for 20 minutes.

3   Heat a large nonstick frying pan over a medium-high heat. Remove the chicken from the marinade, add to the frying pan, and sear for 2 minutes on each side or until golden brown.

4   Scatter the prunes and thyme over the roasted onions and garlic, then pour in the remaining wine and the stock. Place the seared chicken breasts on top and put the pan back in the oven. Bake for 15–20 minutes or until the chicken is cooked through.

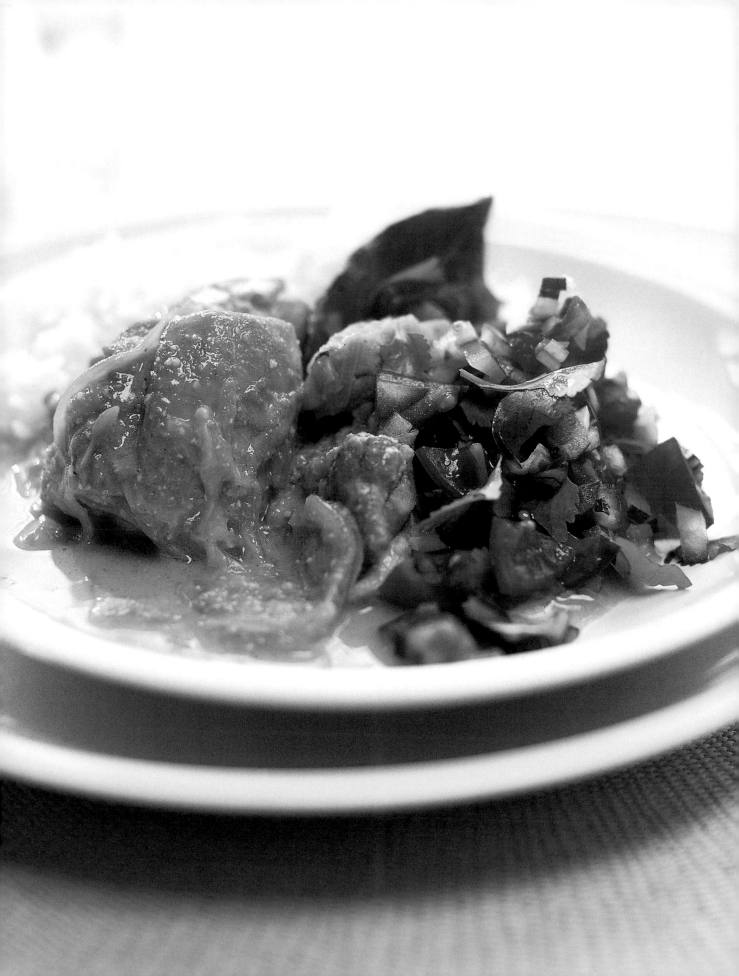

chicken korma

My light version of this popular rich Indian curry is delicious and creamy but much lower in fat. I use reduced-fat coconut milk, plain yogurt, and almonds to enrich the curry. If you want more heat, add dried chili flakes with the spices. Serve the curry with the refreshing relish, and basmati rice or chapattis.

SERVES 4

2 tablespoons sunflower oil

2 large onions, peeled and finely sliced

12 boneless, skinless chicken thighs, halved

3 garlic cloves, peeled and crushed

1 tablespoon garam masala

2 teaspoons ground turmeric

1 bay leaf

2 cups chicken stock

1/3 cup plain yogurt

2/3 cup canned coconut milk (preferably reduced-fat)

2 tablespoons ground almonds

1/4 cup chopped mint leaves

FOR THE RELISH:

4 ripe tomatoes, chopped

1 small red onion, peeled and minced

1/4 cup chopped cilantro

squeeze of lemon juice

freshly ground black pepper

1 Heat 1 tablespoon oil in a large, shallow pan. Add the onions and steam-fry for 10 minutes until softened. Remove the parchment paper and fry for a further 5 minutes until beginning to brown.

2 Meanwhile, heat the remaining oil in a large nonstick frying pan, add the chicken pieces, and sauté for about 2 minutes on each side or until golden.

3 Add the garlic and spices to the onions and fry, stirring, for about 1 minute, then add the sautéed chicken pieces and bay leaf. Pour in the stock and bring to a boil. Simmer gently for 15–20 minutes or until the chicken is cooked.

4 In the meantime, prepare the relish. Combine the tomatoes, red onion, and cilantro in a bowl. Toss to mix, then add lemon juice and black pepper to taste. Set aside.

5 Stir the yogurt, coconut milk, almonds, and mint into the korma. Warm through, but do not boil or the coconut milk will separate. Season to taste, and serve.

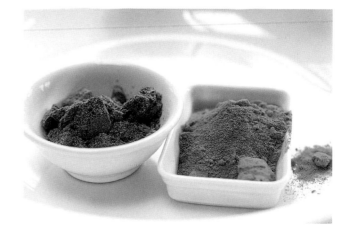

chicken and sesame stir-fry with noodles

This stir-fry is fast, colorful, and packed with nutrients. Broccoli is an important source of vitamins and minerals, including antioxidants that may help to reduce the risk of heart disease and some forms of cancer. Stir-frying helps to preserve the vitamin C content.

SERVES 4

2 large boneless, skinless chicken breast halves
1 tablespoon olive oil
1 garlic clove, peeled and crushed
2-inch piece fresh ginger, peeled and minced
2 cups broccoli florets
2 large carrots
1 bunch of green onions, trimmed

8 oz medium egg noodles
2 tablespoons soy sauce
1 tablespoon honey
juice of 1 orange
1 tablespoon sesame seeds, toasted
freshly ground black pepper

1 Cut the chicken breasts into thin strips and place in a bowl with the olive oil, garlic, and ginger. Toss to mix and set to one side.

2 Put the broccoli florets in a heatproof bowl, cover with boiling water, and let stand for 1 minute. Drain, refresh under cold running water, and drain well. Cut the carrots into thin matchstick strips. Halve the green onions and cut into strips lengthwise.

3 Heat a large nonstick wok or nonstick pan, add the chicken, and stir-fry for 2 minutes. Add the carrots, broccoli, and 1 tablespoon water. Cover with a lid and steam-fry for 4–5 minutes until the chicken is cooked, adding the green onions for the last minute.

4 Meanwhile, cook the noodles according to the package directions. In a bowl, mix together the soy sauce, honey, and orange juice.

5 Drain the noodles thoroughly and add to the pan, along with the soy mixture. Toss until everything is piping hot. Season, and scatter the sesame seeds over the top. Serve at once, in warm bowls.

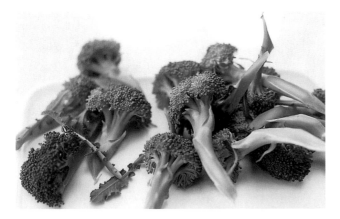

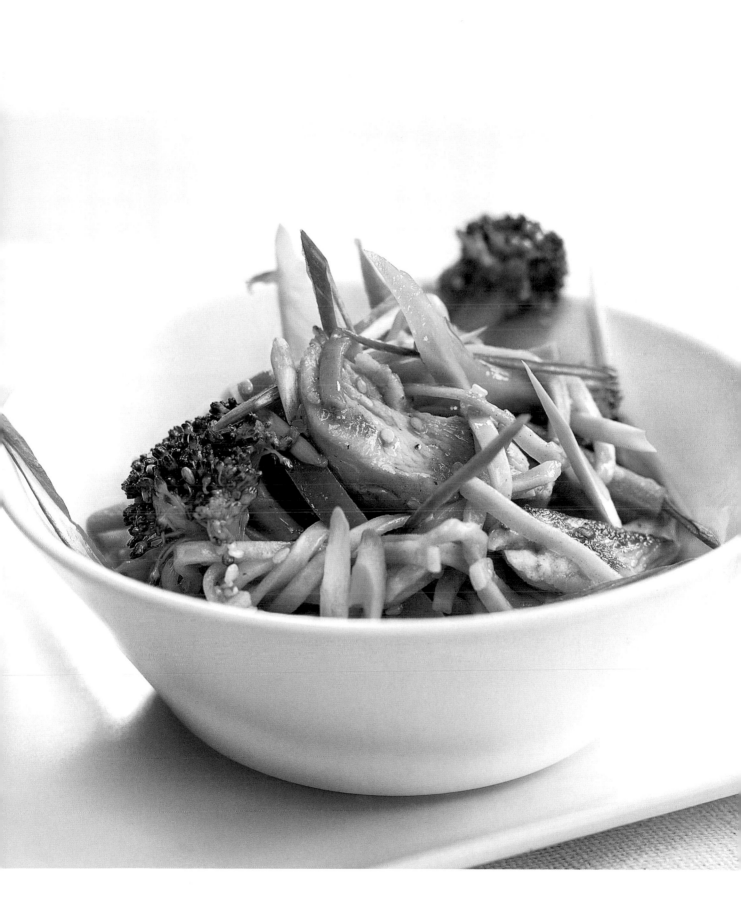

roast chicken and leftovers

A golden bird roasted with the merest drizzle of olive oil, a squeeze of lemon, and some pepper is an unbeatable Sunday lunch. Organic or free-range chickens will give a much better flavor than intensively farmed birds. Simply roast at 400°F for 20 minutes per pound plus an additional 20 minutes, until done (160°F in the breast, 170°F in the thigh). Roast breast-side down for half the cooking time, breast-side up for the remainder. And, for a healthy approach, serve with a fresh fruit salsa or garlicky raita rather than a gravy that's high in fat.

For chicken or turkey breast, oven steaming is an excellent option. Loosely wrap in foil with a splash of wine, a slice of lemon, or some fresh herbs, then cook in the oven at the same temperature for about 20–25 minutes (or longer for turkey) until cooked through. Invariably you'll have meat leftover from a roast for a nourishing soup or the following tasty recipes; each serves 4.

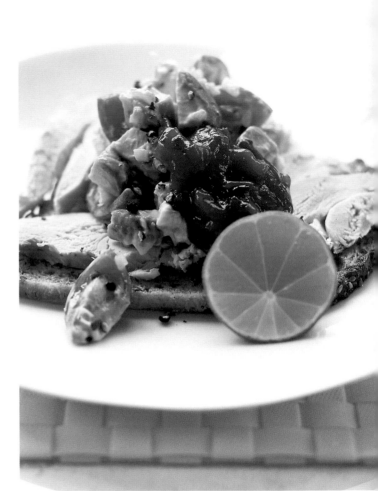

chicken and avocado on rye
Mix the chopped flesh of 1 large, ripe avocado with a squeeze of lime juice, 1 minced shallot, 1 small crushed garlic clove, a dash of Tabasco, 2 tbsp plain yogurt, and 4 quartered cherry tomatoes; season. Top 4 slices of rye bread with 4 slices of cooked chicken or turkey breast. Spoon the avocado mixture on top and finish with a spoonful of rich tomato relish. Serve each open sandwich with a lime wedge.

chicken and artichoke pain bagnes

Cut each of 4 whole-wheat rolls into 3 slices horizontally; toast on both sides, then rub with a halved garlic clove. Thinly slice 8 oz cooked chicken breast and 3 plum tomatoes; quarter 4 roasted artichokes in olive oil. Layer half these ingredients on the bottom of the rolls. Season with pepper and torn basil. Press on the middle slice of each roll and repeat the filling layer. Put on the tops and press down gently.

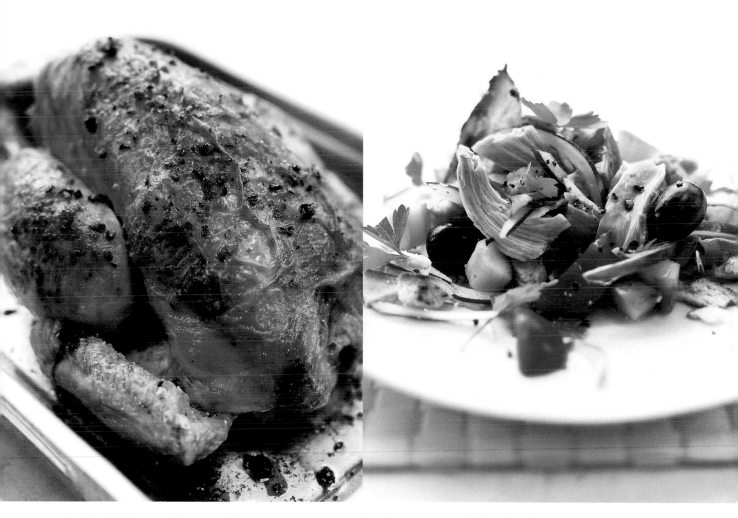

spicy hot chicken and prune subs

Mix 6 tbsp reduced-fat mayonnaise with 6 tbsp plain yogurt and 2 heaped tsp Thai red curry paste in a bowl. Add ½ cup chopped prunes and 1 cup cooked chicken, torn into strips. Mix well; season. In another bowl, toss ½ finely sliced red onion with 4 handfuls of arugula leaves and a large squeeze of lime juice; season. Split 4 submarine rolls and toast, cut-side down, on a hot nonstick grill pan. Fill with the chicken and prune mixture and the arugula salad to serve.

Mediterranean-style bread salad

Toast 3 split white pita breads until crisp. Combine 1½ cups shredded cooked chicken, 1 chopped, seeded hothouse cucumber, 6 quartered small tomatoes, 1 thinly sliced red onion, 20 pitted black olives, and ¼ cup chopped Italian parsley in a bowl. Whisk 2 tbsp extra virgin olive oil with 3 crushed garlic cloves, juice of 1 lemon, and pepper to taste; use to dress the salad. Break the crisp pitas over the salad and toss gently and serve.

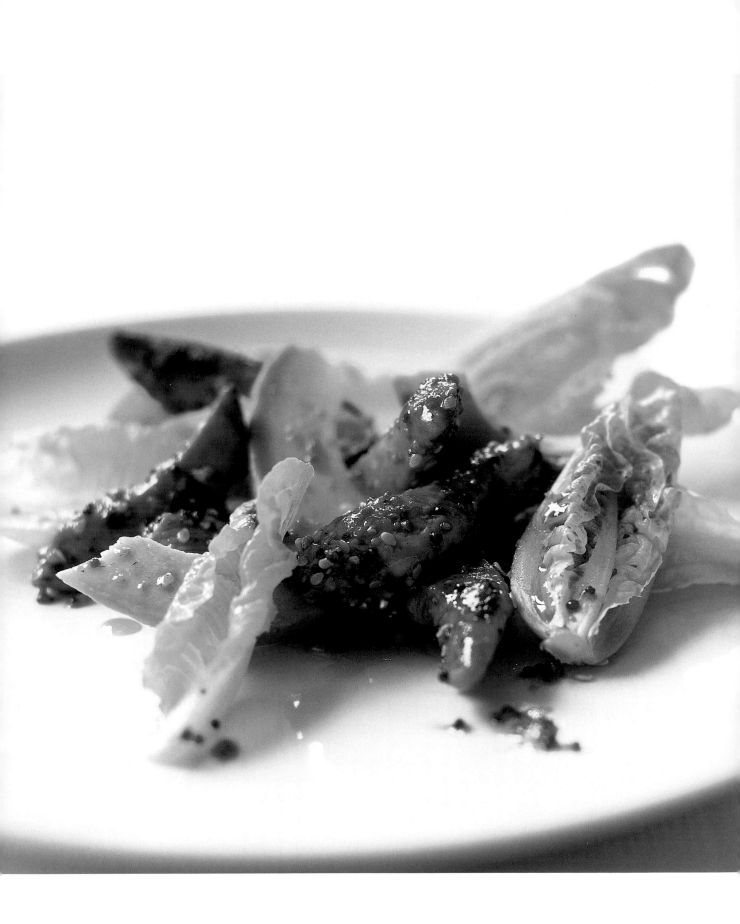

hot sesame chicken and avocado salad

Packed with flavor, this tasty, quick, and easy dish includes my favorite fruit, the avocado. Regarded as a "super food," avocado contains more protein than any other fruit, plenty of vitamin E, and useful potassium. It is also rich in monounsaturated fatty acids, which provide energy and are believed to help maintain a healthy heart. Serve this light, healthy lunch or supper with warm crusty bread to mop up the delicious juices.

SERVES 4

2 large boneless, skinless chicken breast halves

3 tablespoons grain mustard

1 tablespoon honey

juice of 1 lemon

1/2 tablespoon sunflower oil

1 ripe avocado, pitted, peeled, and sliced

2 large handfuls of crisp salad leaves

2 tablespoons sesame seeds

1 teaspoon toasted sesame oil

freshly ground black pepper

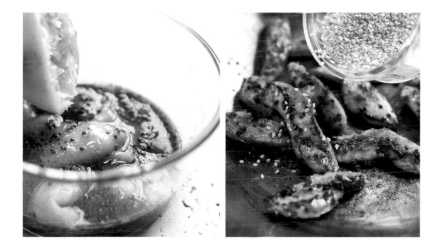

1   Cut the chicken breast halves into finger-sized strips and place in a bowl. Season with black pepper and add the mustard, honey, and lemon juice. Toss the chicken to mix well.

2   Heat the sunflower oil in a nonstick wok or large nonstick frying pan until very hot. Add the chicken mixture and stir-fry for 5–6 minutes or until golden and cooked. Meanwhile, toss the avocado slices with the salad leaves and pile onto four large plates.

3   Add the sesame seeds to the chicken and cook for a further minute or until the seeds are just beginning to color. Spoon the hot sesame chicken on top of the salad leaves, drizzle the sesame oil over, and serve at once.

Thai turkey burgers

These lowfat, high-protein turkey burgers contain naturally sweet grated carrot to keep them moist. Flavored with Thai green curry paste and green onions, the burgers are served in crisp bread rolls with salad leaves and mango chutney.

SERVES 4

1 lb ground turkey
1 heaped cup grated carrots
4 green onions, trimmed and chopped
1¹/₂ tablespoons Thai green curry paste
1 small egg white
1 tablespoon peanut oil
4 large, crisp bread rolls
handful of crisp salad leaves, such as arugula
4 cherry tomatoes, sliced
mango chutney for serving

1 In a large bowl, mix the ground turkey with the grated carrots, green onions, and Thai green curry paste. Add the egg white and stir well to combine.

2 Divide the turkey mixture into four equal portions and shape into burgers. Place on a small board, cover with plastic wrap, and chill for 20 minutes.

3 Heat the peanut oil in a large nonstick frying pan. Add the turkey burgers and cook for 5–6 minutes on each side or until golden and cooked through.

4 Split open the bread rolls. Serve the burgers in the rolls with crisp salad leaves, cherry tomato slices, and a large spoonful of mango chutney.

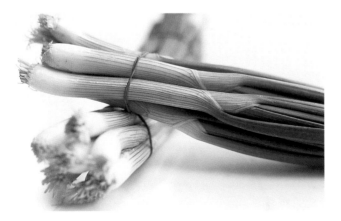

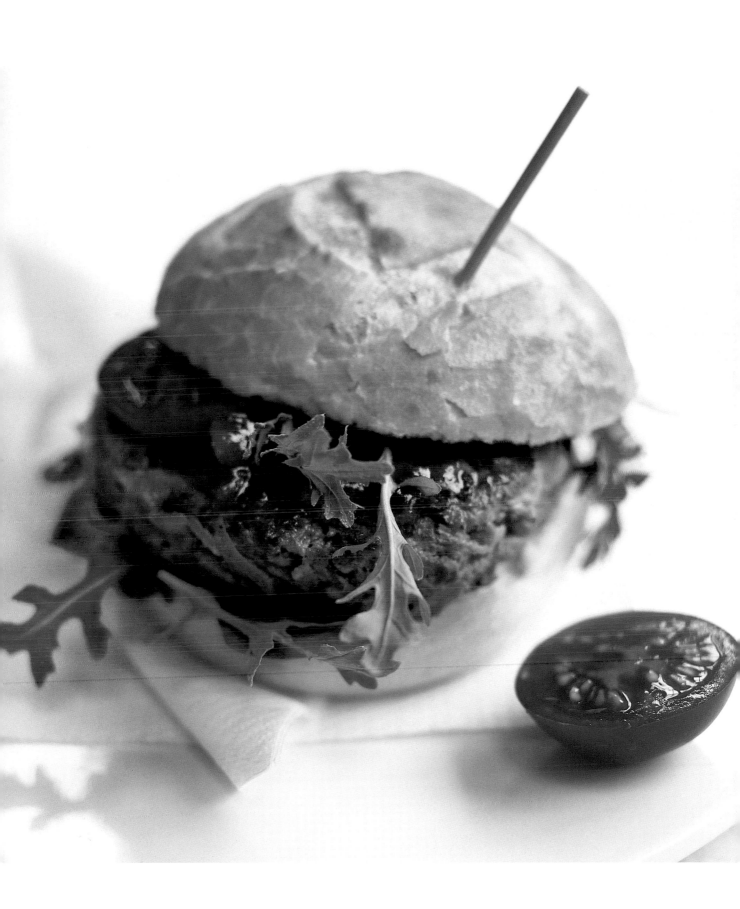

turkey steaks with zesty gremolata

These turkey steaks are simply pan-grilled and finished with an unusual topping of crisp bread crumbs flavored with parsley, lemon, and garlic (called gremolata). Sweet roasted green beans and tomatoes make a delicious accompaniment. Tomatoes are particularly good for you, as they contain vitamins C and E, potassium, and carotenoids, including lycopene, which is an antioxidant that may help to reduce the risk of certain forms of cancer.

SERVES 4

4 turkey steaks, each about 4 oz

grated zest and juice of 1 lemon

2 tablespoons olive oil

1 large sourdough bread roll, coarsely grated

1 garlic clove, peeled and minced

¼ cup chopped Italian parsley

freshly ground black pepper

FOR THE ROASTED BEANS AND TOMATOES:

8 oz baby plum tomatoes

8 oz fine green beans, trimmed

1 Preheat the oven to 400°F. Place each turkey steak between two pieces of plastic wrap or wax paper and beat to a ¼-inch thickness, using a rolling pin. Lay the turkey steaks in a shallow baking dish and pour the lemon juice and 1 tablespoon olive oil over them. Season with pepper.

2 Place the tomatoes and green beans in a roasting pan, drizzle the remaining olive oil over, and season with pepper. Scatter the grated bread in another small roasting pan.

3 Place both roasting pans in the oven. Remove the bread crumbs after 5 minutes; they will be crisp and golden. Continue to cook the beans and tomatoes for a further 8–10 minutes.

4 Meanwhile, heat a ridged nonstick grill pan until very hot. Add the turkey steaks and cook for 2–3 minutes on each side. (You may have to do this in two batches.)

5 Toss the toasted crumbs, lemon zest, garlic, and parsley together in a bowl. Season this gremolata with pepper. Place the turkey steaks on warm serving plates, spoon the roasted beans and tomatoes on top, and finish with a generous scattering of gremolata crumbs. Serve at once.

aromatic turkey pilaf

Bulghur wheat has a good texture and a delicious nutty taste. In this pilaf it takes the place of the more familiar rice. Carrots make a healthy addition, as they are a rich source of beta-carotene, which is converted to vitamin A in the body. Beta-carotene may also boost the immune system and help reduce the risk of some forms of cancer. You can replace the turkey with chicken or lean pork, if you prefer, or, for a meat-free pilaf, finish with a scattering of toasted pine nuts or sliced almonds.

SERVES 4

10 oz skinless, boneless turkey breast
$1^{1}/_{3}$ cups bulghur wheat, rinsed
1 tablespoon sunflower oil
1 large onion, peeled and chopped
1 garlic clove, peeled and crushed
$1^{1}/_{2}$ tablespoons garam masala
1 cup chopped dried apricots
$2/_{3}$ cup golden raisins
1 bay leaf
2 large carrots, peeled and coarsely grated
$2^{1}/_{2}$–3 cups chicken stock
4 tablespoons chopped cilantro
freshly ground black pepper
1 large lemon, cut into wedges, for serving

1   Cut the turkey into $1/_{2}$-inch slices and set aside. Put the bulghur wheat in a bowl and add enough cold water to cover generously. Let stand for 15 minutes.

2   Meanwhile, heat the oil in a large nonstick sauté pan or nonstick wok, add the onion, and cook for 5 minutes until softened. Increase the heat and add the turkey. Fry, turning frequently, for 3–4 minutes or until the turkey is golden all over. Stir in the garlic and garam masala, and cook for a further minute.

3   Add the dried fruits, bay leaf, and grated carrots, then pour in $2^{1}/_{2}$ cups of stock. Drain the bulghur wheat and add to the pan. Season with black pepper. Cover and cook gently for 15 minutes. Add extra stock if the pilaf becomes too dry; it should have the consistency of a risotto.

4   Spoon the pilaf into a large serving dish and stir in the cilantro, reserving a tablespoon to scatter over the top. Serve with the lemon wedges.

5 meat

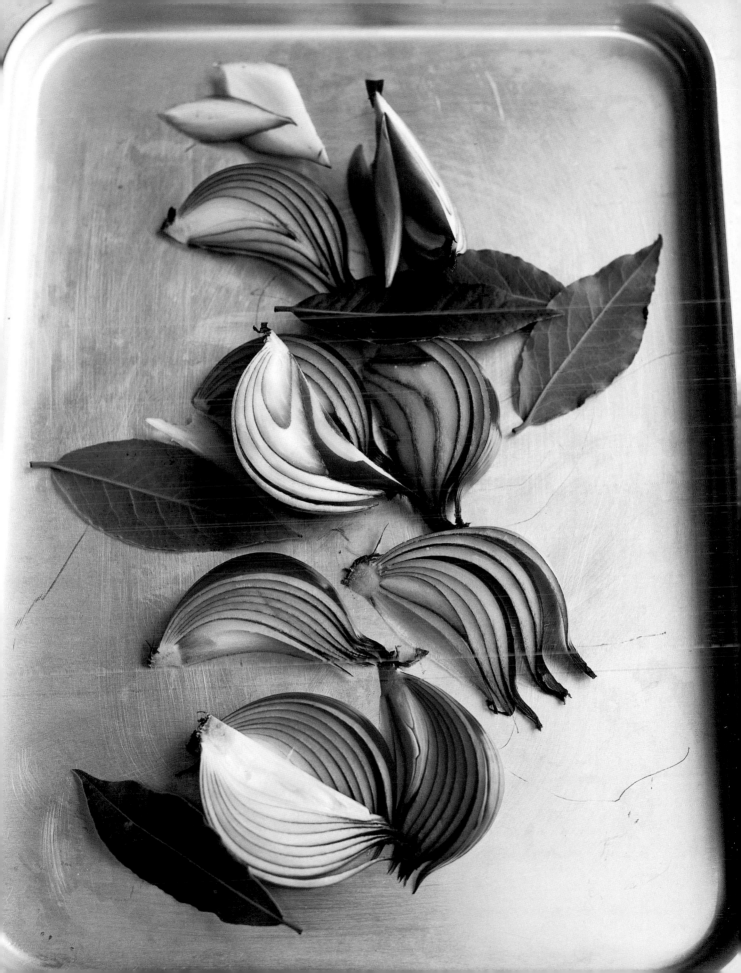

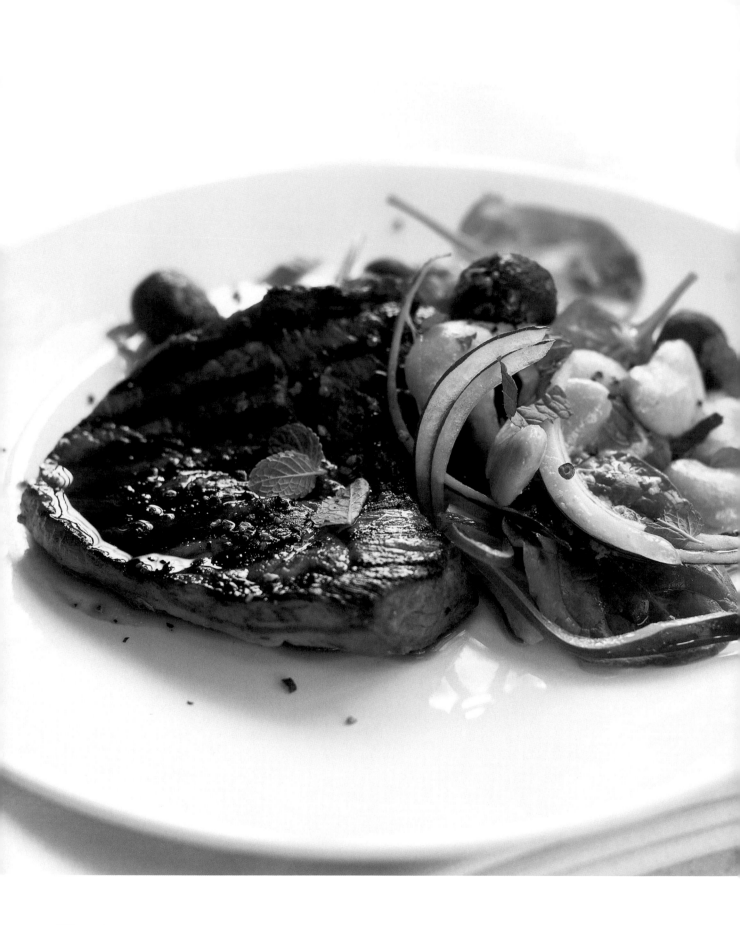

lamb steaks with minted beet and spinach salad

Lean lamb steaks are pan-grilled and served with a salad of baby spinach, lima beans, and baby beets in a fresh minty dressing. Lima beans provide slow-release carbohydrate, and spinach is a good source of minerals and vitamins.

SERVES 4

4 lamb leg steaks, each about 5 oz
2 garlic cloves, peeled and crushed
2 tablespoons balsamic vinegar
1 tablespoon olive oil
1¹/₂ cups baby spinach leaves
14 oz canned baby lima beans, drained and
  rinsed
1 red onion, peeled and thinly sliced
8 oz fresh baby beets, cooked and peeled
freshly ground black pepper
FOR THE DRESSING:
1 tablespoon olive oil
1 tablespoon white wine vinegar
1 teaspoon Dijon mustard
pinch of sugar
¹/₄ cup chopped mint

1 Place the lamb steaks in a non-metallic bowl. Add the garlic, balsamic vinegar, 1 tablespoon olive oil, and plenty of black pepper. Turn the lamb steaks in the marinade to coat well, then set aside in the refrigerator for at least 20 minutes.

2 To make the dressing, whisk the olive oil, wine vinegar, mustard, sugar, and mint together in a large bowl. Season with a little black pepper. Set aside.

3 Heat a nonstick grill pan over a medium-high heat. Add the lamb and cook for 2–3 minutes each side for medium rare or longer to your liking. Pour in the marinade, and bubble and reduce to a glaze for the lamb steaks.

4 Meanwhile, add the spinach, lima beans, and red onion to the dressing and toss gently to combine. Divide the salad among four large serving plates. Dot with the baby beets and serve immediately with the lamb steaks.

babotie burgers

There's nothing better than homemade burgers, and these South African-style lamb burgers are particularly good. The fruity apple and mango relish is the ideal complement.

SERVES 4 (OR 8)

4 teaspoons olive oil
1 large onion, peeled and minced
1 tablespoon garam masala
1 teaspoon ground cinnamon
1 lb ground lamb
1 large carrot, peeled and grated
1 1/2 cups fresh white bread crumbs
1/2 cup chopped almonds

grated zest of 1 lemon
1 egg, beaten
freshly ground black pepper

FOR THE RELISH:

1/3 cup golden raisins
2 crisp apples, diced
1 tablespoon hot (spicy) mango chutney
seeds of 6 cardamom pods, crushed
2 tablespoons chopped mint

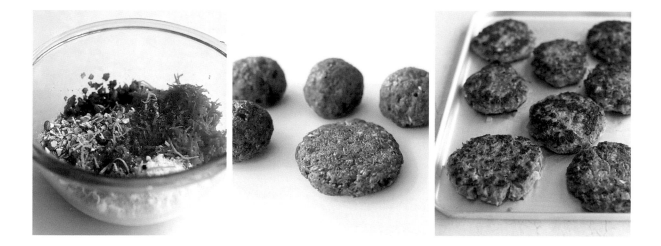

1 Preheat the oven to 350°F. Heat 2 teaspoons of the olive oil in a pan and gently fry the onion for 10 minutes until soft and golden. Add the garam masala and cinnamon, and cook for a further minute. Tip into a large bowl and let cool.

2 Add the ground lamb, grated carrot, bread crumbs, chopped almonds, and lemon zest to the cooled spiced onion and mix well. Season with pepper and add the beaten egg to bind the mixture.

3 Divide the mixture into eight portions. Roll into balls, then flatten to make small burgers. Heat the remaining olive oil in a large, nonstick frying pan and sear the burgers quickly on each side.

4 Place the seared burgers on a nonstick baking sheet and put into the oven to bake for 10–15 minutes or until cooked through. Meanwhile, mix all the ingredients for the relish together and season to taste. Serve the burgers with the fruit relish, crusty bread, and a leaf salad.

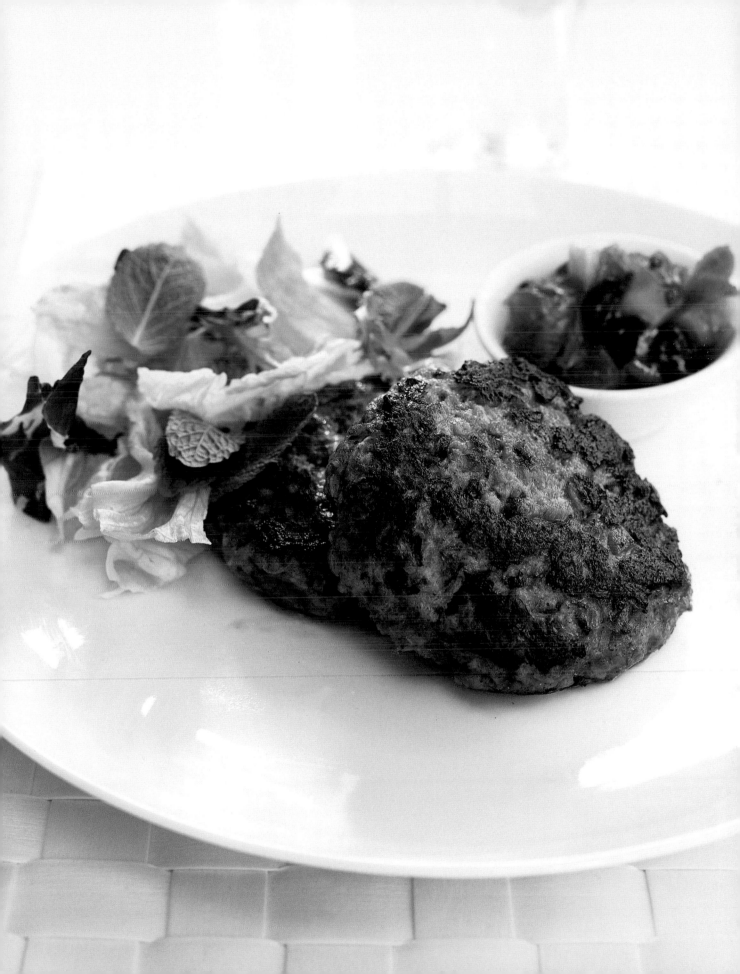

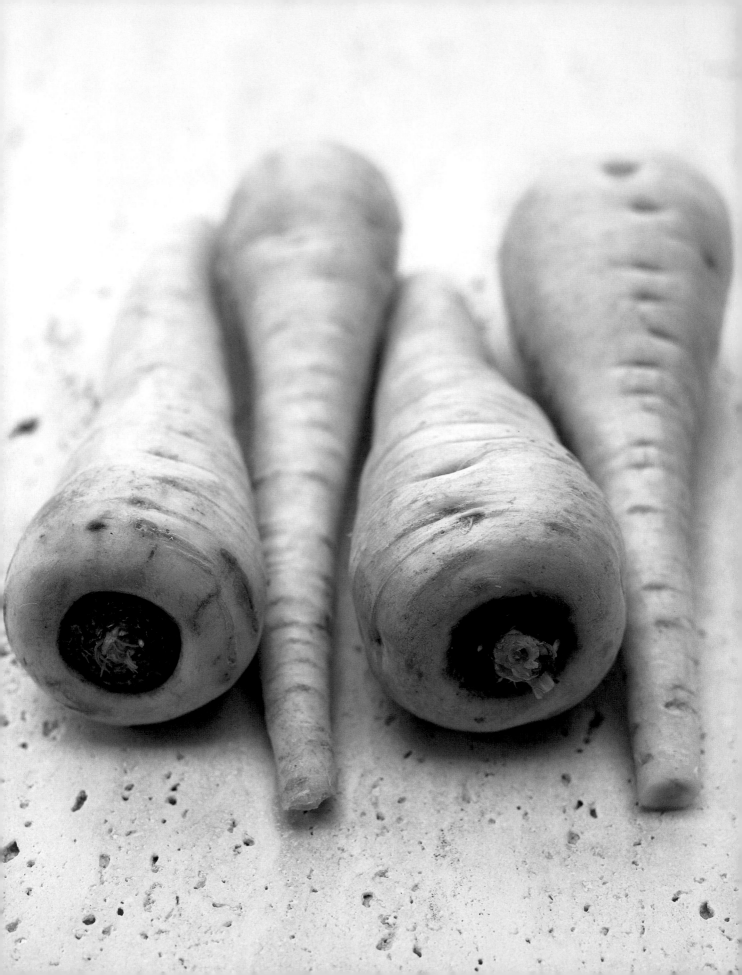

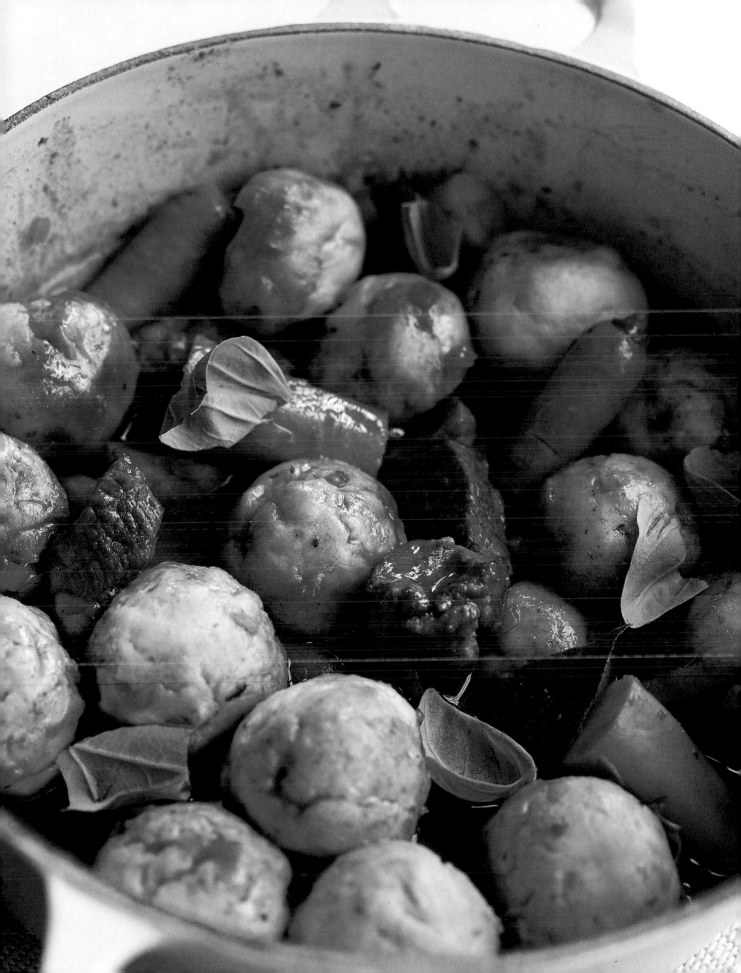

lamb and parsnip ragout

This is real comfort food—a rich lamb stew with whole baby carrots and parsnip chunks, topped with gnocchi. It's a lighter, healthier version of a classic stew with dumplings. Experiment with the gnocchi by using different flavors, such as garlic and thyme, or chili and chives, sprinkling the stew with thyme or chives before serving. *Illustrated on page 113*

SERVES 4

12 oz lean boneless leg of lamb
1 tablespoon all-purpose flour
1 tablespoon olive oil
1 onion, peeled and minced
8 baby carrots, trimmed and scrubbed
2 parsnips, peeled and cut into chunks
2 bay leaves
2 tablespoons tomato paste
1¼ cups red wine
2 cups vegetable stock
2 tablespoons torn basil
freshly ground black pepper

FOR THE GARLIC GNOCCHI:

1²/₃ cups all-purpose flour
1 teaspoon baking powder
2 garlic cloves, peeled and crushed
2 tablespoons olive oil
½ cup milk

1 Cut the lamb into ¾-inch chunks and toss in the seasoned flour. Heat the oil in a large, shallow, heavy pan and fry the lamb over a high heat until browned all over. Remove with a slotted spoon and set aside.

2 Add 2 tablespoons water and the onion to the pan. Stir well over a medium heat, scraping up the crusty golden bits from the bottom of the pan. Lower the heat, cover, and steam-fry for 5 minutes, stirring occasionally.

3 Stir in the carrots, parsnips, and bay leaves, and cook for 2 minutes. Return the lamb to the pan. Stir in the tomato paste, red wine, and stock. Bring to a boil, then cover and simmer for 25–30 minutes or until the lamb and vegetables are just tender.

4 To make the gnocchi, sift the flour and baking powder into a bowl and season well. Make a well in the middle. Mix together the garlic, olive oil, and milk, and add to the well. Gradually incorporate the flour to make a soft but not sticky dough.

5 Shape the dough into 16 small rounds and arrange on top of the ragout. Replace the lid and simmer for a further 10 minutes. Scatter the basil over the ragout just before serving.

steak and mushroom rolls with mustard sauce

Pan-grilled steak strips are served in toasted petit pains with meaty mushrooms, peppery, iron-rich watercress, and a creamy mustard sauce, for a satisfying supper or lunch. Lean beef is a good source of easily absorbed iron and is also rich in zinc. Always let steak rest before cutting, as this allows the juices to be reabsorbed and keeps the meat really succulent.

SERVES 4

2 portobello mushrooms
4 teaspoons olive oil
12 oz boneless sirloin steak
1 teaspoon Worcestershire sauce
4 petit pains (French bread rolls) or other crusty
   bread rolls
1¹/₂ cups watercress
freshly ground black pepper
FOR THE MUSTARD SAUCE:
2 tablespoons crème fraîche or light sour cream
1 tablespoon Dijon mustard
1 tablespoon grain mustard

1 Preheat the broiler. Brush the mushrooms with 3 teaspoons of the oil and season with black pepper. Broil for 6 minutes on each side or until just cooked.

2 To make the sauce, mix the crème fraîche or sour cream with the Dijon and grain mustards in a small bowl until evenly blended. Set aside.

3 Preheat a nonstick grill pan until very hot. Brush the steak with the Worcestershire sauce and the remaining olive oil, then season with pepper. Place on the grill pan and sear for 2–3 minutes each side or until cooked to your liking. Remove to a warm plate, cover with foil, and let rest for 5 minutes.

4 Cut each bread roll in half and toast the cut sides under the broiler for 1–2 minutes. Thinly slice the steak and mushrooms on the diagonal. Place the watercress on the bottom half of each roll and top with the steak and mushroom slices. Drizzle the mustard sauce over the top and cover with the lid of the roll. Serve immediately.

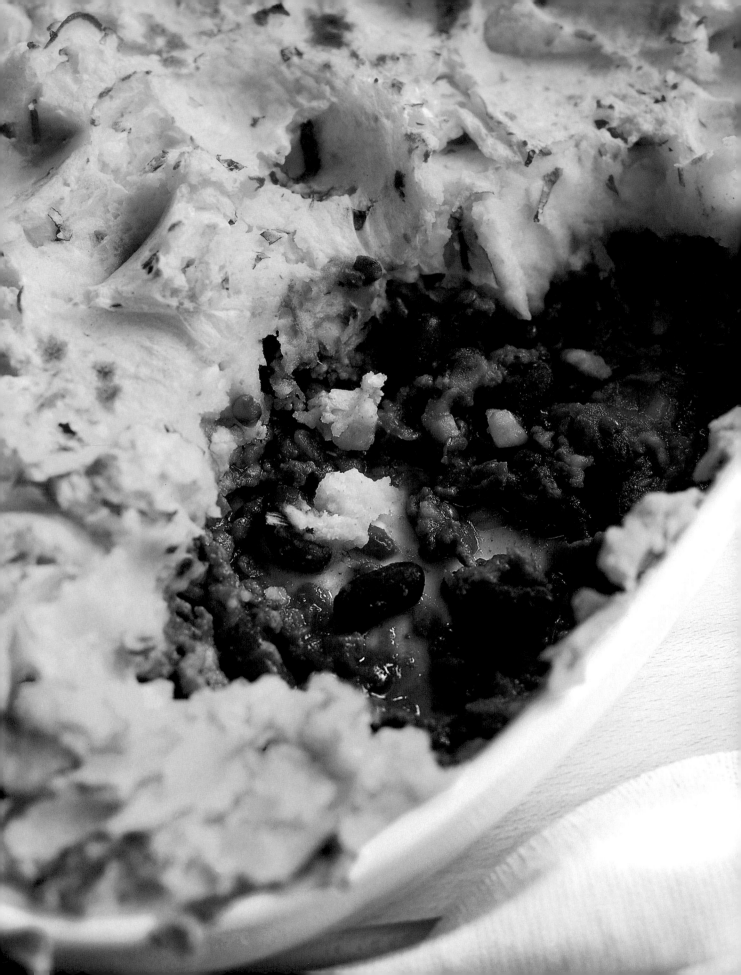

chile con carne pie

You can make this chile as hot as you like. I've used less meat than is usual, and added lentils and beans. The turmeric- and cilantro-flavored mashed potato crust makes a tasty change from the typical chile accompaniment of rice. A little chocolate added at the end, Mexican-style, really enhances the color and flavor.

SERVES 4–6

1 tablespoon olive oil

1 onion, peeled and minced

1 garlic clove, peeled and crushed

9 oz ground round or other lean ground beef

2 hot red chili peppers, seeded and minced

1 teaspoon ground cumin

1 tablespoon tomato paste

14 oz canned crushed tomatoes

1¼ cups vegetable stock

½ cup lentils

14 oz canned red kidney beans, drained and rinsed

½ oz (½ square) bittersweet chocolate, roughly chopped

freshly ground black pepper

FOR THE CRUST:

2 lb all-purpose potatoes, peeled

3 tablespoons hot lowfat milk

1 teaspoon ground turmeric

2 tablespoons chopped cilantro

1 Heat the olive oil in a large pan, add the onion and garlic, and cook for 5 minutes. Turn up the heat, add the beef, and cook, stirring, for 3 minutes or until browned. Stir in the chili peppers and cumin, and cook for 1 minute.

2 Add the tomato paste, crushed tomatoes, stock, lentils, and kidney beans. Bring to a boil, then simmer for 25–30 minutes. Stir in the chocolate and season with black pepper.

3 Meanwhile, for the crust, cut the potatoes into even-sized chunks, put into a pan of cold water, and bring to a boil. Simmer for 20 minutes or until tender, then drain. Tip the potatoes back into the pan and mash over a low heat, stirring in the milk, turmeric, and cilantro. Season to taste.

4 Preheat the broiler. Spoon the chile into a gratin or baking dish and spread the hot mashed potatoes roughly over the top. Place under the broiler for 5 minutes or until the topping is crisp and golden brown.

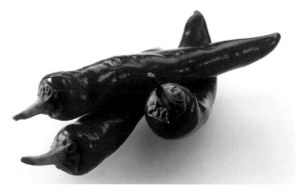

gingered beef curry

A really light, quick curry, this is cooked in a novel way. Lean, tender sirloin steak is pan-grilled to remain juicy and pink, then set aside to rest. Chick peas soak up the spicy flavors of the curry sauce, and shredded greens and the steak strips are added at the end of cooking. Serve the curry on its own, or with basmati rice or chapattis.

SERVES 4

1¼ lb boneless sirloin steaks
1 tablespoon olive oil
2 onions, peeled and sliced
2 tablespoons Madras curry paste
2-inch piece fresh ginger, peeled and grated
2½ cups vegetable stock
14 oz canned chick peas (garbanzo beans),
  drained and rinsed
1 cup finely shredded hearty greens such as kale
  or Savoy cabbage
freshly ground black pepper

1   Brush the steaks with a little olive oil and sprinkle with coarsely ground black pepper. Heat a nonstick grill pan until very hot. Add the steaks to the grill pan and sear for 2 minutes on each side for medium rare, or 1–2 minutes longer according to taste. Set aside to rest.

2   Heat the remaining olive oil in a large shallow pan, add the onions, and cook over a gentle heat for 5 minutes until beginning to soften. Add the curry paste to the pan and stir well. Cover and steam-fry for 5 minutes over a medium heat, stirring occasionally. Stir in the ginger and cook for 2 minutes.

3   Add the stock and chick peas to the pan, stir well, and bring to a boil. Simmer for 10 minutes. Stir in the greens, cover, and cook for a further minute.

4   Slice the steaks into thin strips on the diagonal and stir into the curry. Heat through for 1 minute, and season to taste before serving.

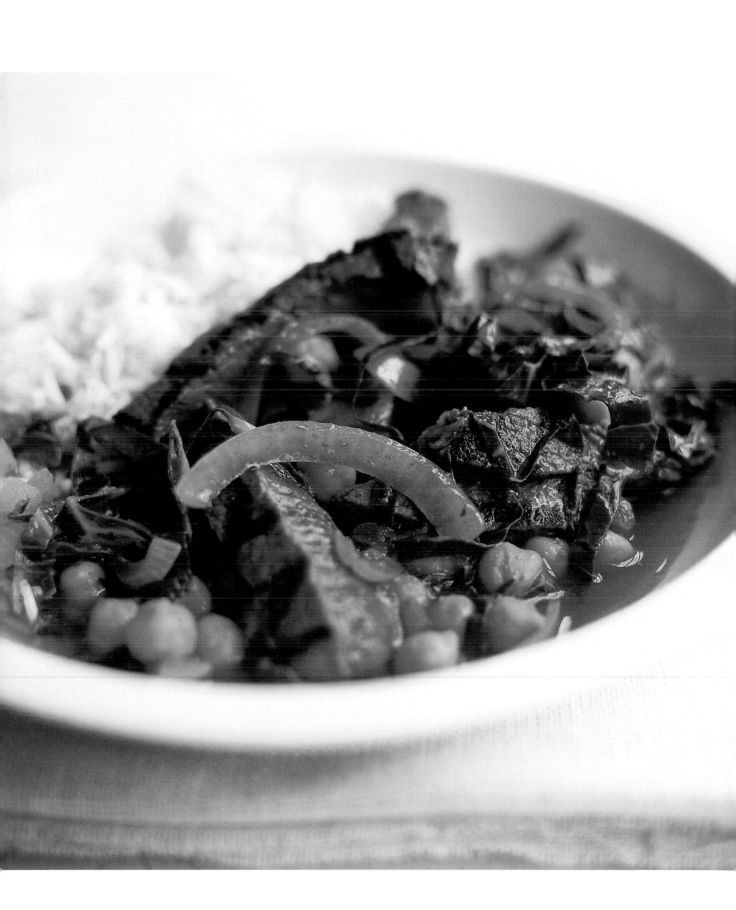

a little meat goes a long way

For most people, red meat is one of the main sources of protein and a good source of iron. But you don't need to consume as much as you may think. An average adult needs just 3 ounces of protein per day—that is about as much as you can hold in the palm of your hand. So the trick is to buy smaller amounts of the best quality meat.

Choose the leanest cuts, such as pork tenderloin, lamb leg, and beef sirloin, and trim away any fat. Look for very lean ground beef and bind it with an egg white and a dash of Worcestershire sauce to make your own burgers—then you'll know exactly what's in them! Lean cuts of meat are ideal pan-grilled, broiled, grilled, stir- or steam-fried, and roasted. Use meat as a flavoring rather than the main ingredient in a dish, by combining it with lots of vegetables or salad, and you will appreciate its flavor and goodness in the best possible way. Each of the following recipes serves 4.

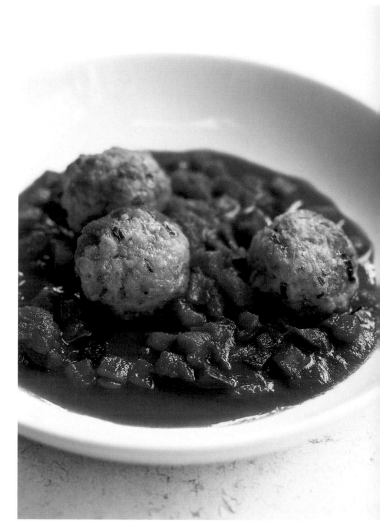

pork meatballs with goulash sauce
Mix 12 oz lean ground pork, 1 cup grated carrot, the grated zest of 2 lemons, ¼ cup diced sun-dried tomatoes, 2 tbsp chopped chives, 2 cups fresh white bread crumbs, 1 medium egg white, and pepper to taste. Shape into 12 balls. Bake at 400°F for 15 minutes or until cooked. Sauté 2 diced eggplants in 1 tbsp oil for 5 minutes. Add 2 tsp smoked paprika and cook for 30 seconds. Stir in 1½ cups tomato sauce and 1 cup red wine. Simmer for 5 minutes. Serve with the meatballs.

steak salad with hot green sauce

Toss 4 red onions, in wedges, in 1 tbsp olive oil and bake at 400°F for 35 minutes. Sear an 8-oz filet mignon all over on a smoking nonstick grill pan for 4–5 minutes. Rest for 5 minutes. Toss the onions with 14 oz canned green lentils, drained and rinsed, 1 bunch watercress, 1 tbsp olive oil, and pepper to taste. Mix 1 tbsp wasabi paste with ½ cup plain yogurt. Slice the steak and serve on the salad. Top with the wasabi dressing.

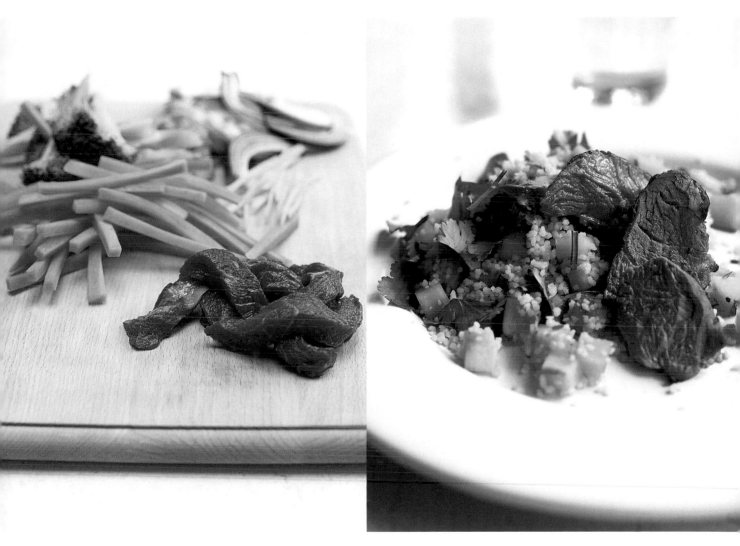

sticky beef and bok choy stir-fry

Cook 9 oz fine egg noodles. Heat 2 tsp peanut oil in a nonstick wok and stir-fry 8 oz sirloin steak strips over high heat for 2 minutes. Add 1 bunch minced green onions, 2 chopped red bell peppers, 2 crushed garlic cloves, and 4 cups finely shredded bok choy. Stir-fry for 1 minute. Stir in 4 tbsp plum sauce and 2 tbsp dry sherry; bubble for 1 minute. Drain the egg noodles and toss with 2 tsp toasted sesame oil. Serve the peppered beef on lettuce leaves, with the hot noodles.

peppered lamb with nectarine and cumin couscous

Brush 4 lamb leg steaks, 5 oz each, with 2 tsp olive oil and sprinkle with cracked pepper. Soak 1 cup couscous in 1 cup boiling water for 5 minutes. Add 3 tbsp extra virgin olive oil, juice of 1 lemon, pepper, and 2 tsp toasted cumin seeds. Fork through, and add 2 chopped nectarines and ¼ cup chopped cilantro. Heat a nonstick grill pan until smoking. Add the lamb steaks and cook for 6–7 minutes, turning to brown on all sides. Rest for 5 minutes, then slice thinly. Serve with the couscous.

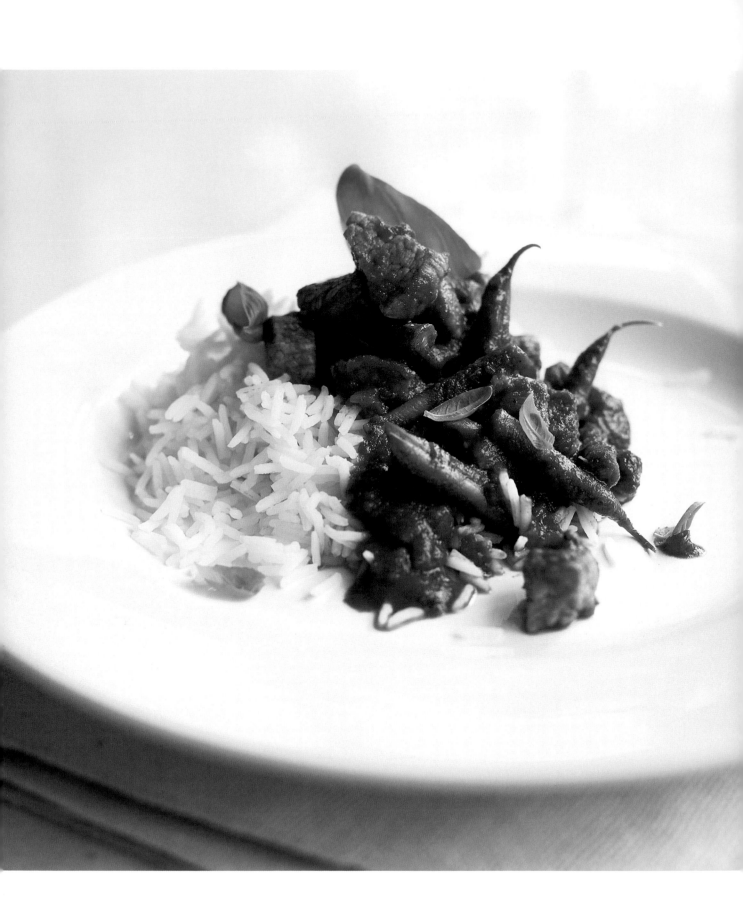

red Thai pork with green beans

For this simple, aromatic curry, lean pork tenderloin is flavored with Thai red curry paste and cooked in tomato purée with green beans. Serve with Thai fragrant rice, and a big dollop of cooling plain yogurt.

SERVES 4

2 teaspoons olive oil

1 red onion, peeled and minced

8-oz pork tenderloin

2 tablespoons Thai red curry paste

2 cups tomato purée

1 teaspoon sugar

12 oz fine green beans, trimmed

freshly ground black pepper

cilantro or small basil leaves for garnish

1 Heat the oil in a large shallow pan, add the red onion, and cook over a gentle heat for 10 minutes until soft and golden.

2 Meanwhile, cut the pork into ¼-inch pieces. Turn up the heat under the pan to high, add the pork, and cook, stirring, for 2 minutes until evenly colored.

3 Stir in the Thai curry paste and cook for 1 minute. Pour in the tomato purée, add the sugar, and stir well. Bring to a boil, then lower the heat and gently simmer for 8 minutes.

4 Meanwhile, blanch the green beans in boiling water for 1 minute. Drain and refresh under cold water; drain again and cut into short lengths. Add the beans to the curry and cook for a further minute.

5 Season with pepper to taste. Scatter cilantro or basil leaves over the curry and serve accompanied by Thai fragrant rice, and yogurt, if desired.

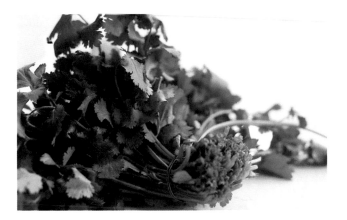

pork koftas with roasted red pepper salad

These spiced, lean pork skewers are served on a mouthwatering salad of roasted bell peppers and arugula, with a piquant sauce. Red bell peppers are one of the best sources of vitamin C.

SERVES 4

3 large red bell peppers, halved, cored, and
  seeded
2 tablespoons olive oil
1 onion, peeled and minced
1 teaspoon cayenne pepper
2 teaspoons ground cumin
2 teaspoons ground coriander
1 lb lean ground pork
1 egg white

$^1/_2$ bunch of Italian parsley, roughly chopped
2 handfuls arugula leaves
freshly ground black pepper
FOR THE SAUCE:
1 cup thick plain yogurt
1 garlic clove, peeled and crushed
$^1/_3$ cup chopped black and green olives
$^1/_2$ bunch of Italian parsley, roughly chopped
squeeze of lemon juice

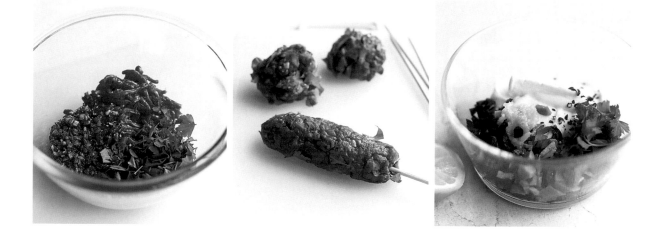

1 Preheat the oven to 400°F. Cut each pepper half into 4 strips, place in a roasting pan, and drizzle 1 tablespoon oil over them. Roast for 35–40 minutes until softened and lightly charred.

2 Meanwhile, heat the remaining olive oil in a pan. Add the onion and cook for 5–6 minutes until softened. Add the spices and cook for a further minute. Transfer to a large bowl and let cool for 5 minutes. Add the ground pork, egg white, parsley, and plenty of black pepper. Mix thoroughly.

3 Preheat the broiler. Divide the pork mixture into eight and shape each into a thick sausage. Push the sharp end of a soaked bamboo skewer through the length of each sausage and place on a broiler pan. Broil the koftas for about 6 minutes, turning occasionally, until cooked through.

4 Meanwhile, combine the sauce ingredients in a bowl; season with pepper. Toss the roasted peppers with the arugula and divide among four plates. Top with the koftas, add a spoonful of sauce, and serve.

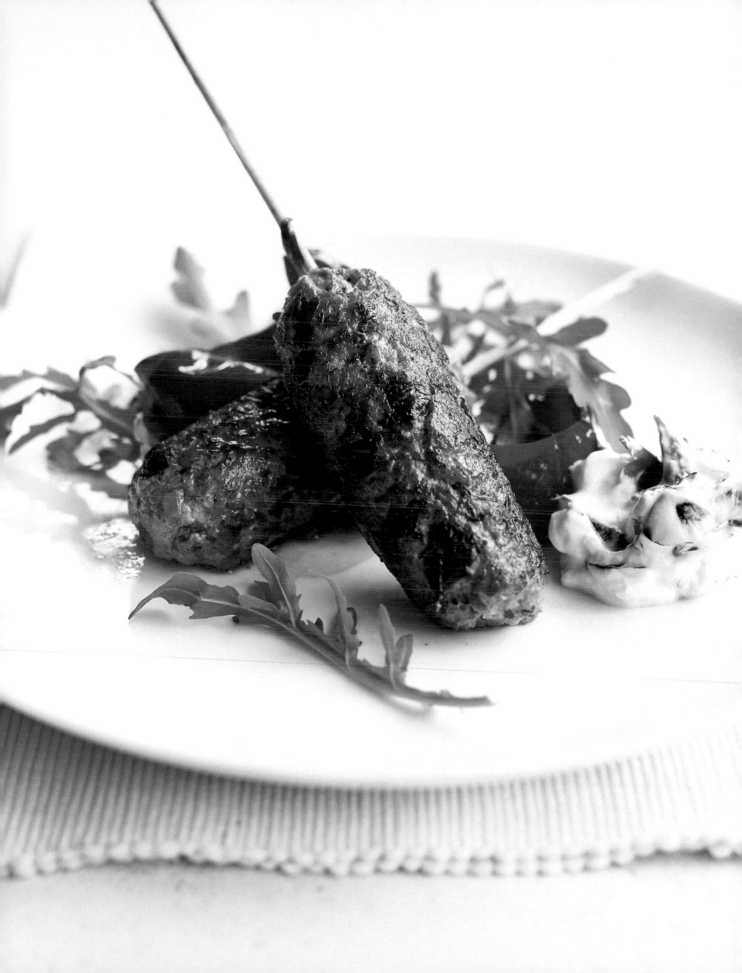

pork and prune tagine-style

This quick version of a Moroccan-style stew is subtly spiced with harissa, a chili paste that features strongly in Middle Eastern cooking. Carrots and prunes give the dish a hint of sweetness plus added nutrients. Carrots are, of course, rich in beta-carotene, the plant form of vitamin A, while prunes are a good source of potassium, iron, and fiber.

SERVES 4

1-lb pork tenderloin, trimmed
2 tablespoons harissa paste
1 tablespoon olive oil
2 cups vegetable stock
1 onion, peeled and thinly sliced
grated zest and juice of 1 orange
4 carrots, peeled and cut into chunks on the
    diagonal
1 cup prunes
1 cinnamon stick
2 tablespoons chopped cilantro
freshly ground black pepper

1 Cut the pork tenderloin across into ½-inch rounds and place in a bowl. Add the harissa paste and toss well to coat evenly.

2 Heat the olive oil in a large shallow pan, add the pork, and cook for 1 minute on each side or until golden. Remove with a slotted spoon and set aside.

3 Add 4 tablespoons of the stock and the onion to the pan, cover, and steam-fry over a medium heat for 5 minutes, stirring occasionally, until softened and golden.

4 Stir in the grated orange zest and juice with the remaining stock. Return the pork to the pan and add the carrots, prunes, and cinnamon stick. Bring to a boil, then lower the heat and simmer for 15–20 minutes.

5 Season to taste with black pepper and scatter the chopped cilantro over the top. Serve the tagine with couscous or basmati rice.

glazed ham with grilled pineapple and corn

Here is a healthy, fresh twist to an old favorite. Lean ham steaks, or pork loin steaks, are marinated in honey and orange juice, pan-grilled, and served with grilled fresh pineapple and baby corn. The marinade is spiked with chili pepper and drizzled over the ham to serve. This is an excellent recipe to boost your vitamin levels and contribute to your five-a-day fruit and veggies.

SERVES 4

4 ham steaks or pork loin steaks, each 5 oz
juice of 2 oranges
1 tablespoon honey
$1/2$ bunch of green onions, trimmed and minced
1 small pineapple
7 oz baby corn
2 teaspoons olive oil
1 hot red chili pepper, seeded and minced
freshly ground black pepper

1   Place the ham steaks in a non-metallic dish, drizzle the orange juice and honey over them, and sprinkle with the green onions. Season well with black pepper. Set aside for 15 minutes.

2   Cut away the skin from the pineapple, then remove the core from each wedge. Heat a nonstick grill pan until really hot. Pan-grill the pineapple wedges and baby corn for 2 minutes each side or until slightly charred on the outside. Remove from the pan and keep warm.

3   Heat the olive oil in the grill pan. Remove the ham steaks from the marinade, reserving the liquid, and add to the pan. Cook for 3–4 minutes on each side, then transfer to warm serving plates.

4   Pour the reserved marinade into the pan and bubble over a medium heat for 1 minute. Stir in the chili pepper and season to taste. Arrange the pineapple and baby corn alongside the ham steaks. Drizzle the hot dressing over and serve.

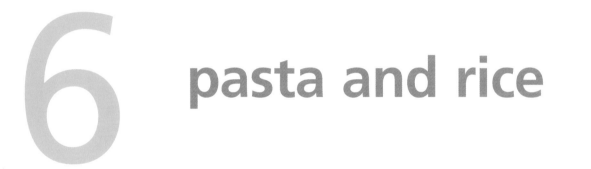

6 pasta and rice

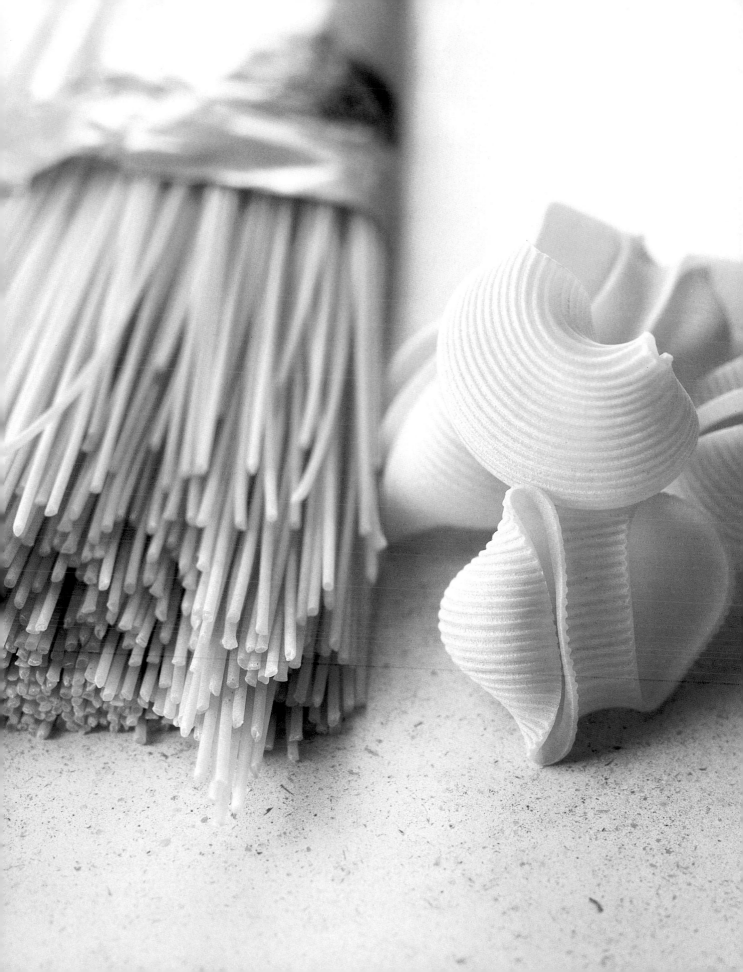

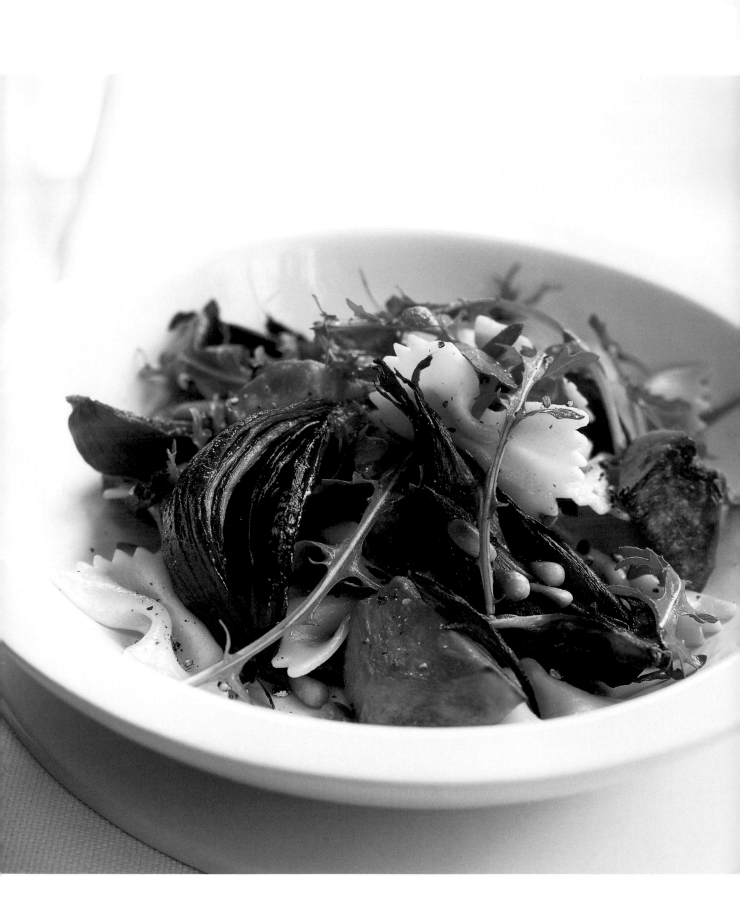

roasted butternut farfalle

Butternut squash and red onion wedges are roasted together until caramelized and sweet, then teamed with arugula, pasta, and toasted pine nuts for a simple, yet stunning and satisfying meal. Winter squash varieties, such as butternut, contain useful amounts of vitamin A.

SERVES 4

1 large butternut squash, peeled, halved, and
  seeded
2 large red onions, peeled and cut into thin
  wedges
2 tablespoons olive oil
12 oz farfalle or other pasta shapes
1/3 cup pine nuts, lightly toasted
2 handfuls of arugula
freshly ground black pepper
balsamic vinegar, for drizzling

1 Preheat the oven to 400°F. Cut the butternut squash into 1-inch pieces and place in a large roasting pan with the red onions. Drizzle the olive oil over and season with black pepper. Roast for 40–45 minutes until the vegetables are tender and slightly caramelized.

2 About 10 minutes before the end of the roasting time, cook the pasta in a large pan of boiling water according to the package directions, until *al dente* (cooked but still a bit firm to the bite).

3 Drain the pasta, reserving 2 tablespoons of the cooking water, then return to the pan. Add the roasted vegetables, pine nuts, and arugula along with the reserved water. Toss to mix and season with plenty of black pepper. Pile onto warm serving plates, drizzle a little balsamic vinegar over, and serve.

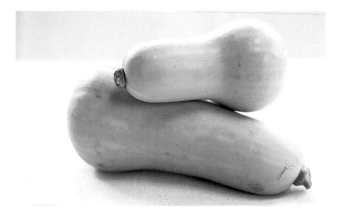

spaghetti rosti with tuna

This is a novel way of serving spaghetti, which is always a favorite in our home. Select tuna packed in water rather than oil or brine. Tuna is an excellent source of protein, although it isn't high in the beneficial omega-3 fatty acids like fresh tuna. Serve the rosti warm, cold, or even cut into wedges and packed into lunchboxes.

SERVES 4–6

8 oz spaghetti

1 tablespoon olive oil

1 onion, peeled and minced

1 garlic clove, peeled and crushed

5 eggs, beaten

14 oz canned white-meat tuna in water,
   drained and flaked

1/3 cup grated sharp cheddar cheese

freshly ground black pepper

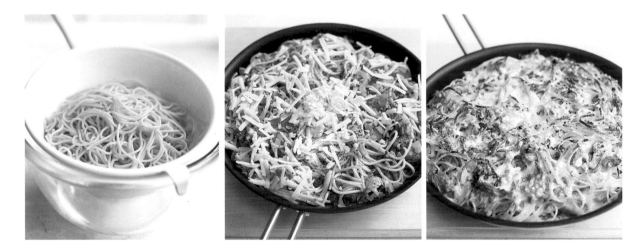

1 Cook the spaghetti in a large pan of boiling water for 8–10 minutes or until *al dente* (cooked but still firm to the bite). Drain, rinse under cold running water, drain well again, and place in a large bowl.

2 Meanwhile, heat the oil in a large nonstick frying pan (suitable for use under the broiler). Add the onion and cook for 5 minutes, then stir in the garlic and cook for a further minute. Add to the cooked pasta with the beaten eggs and tuna, and toss to mix. Season well.

3 Preheat the broiler. Spread the spaghetti mixture evenly in the frying pan and scatter the cheese over the top. Cook over a medium heat for 10 minutes or until the eggs are almost set.

4 Place under the broiler and cook for 3–4 minutes or until just set and golden on top. Slide the rosti out of the pan onto a board. Cut into wedges and serve with roasted tomatoes or salad leaves.

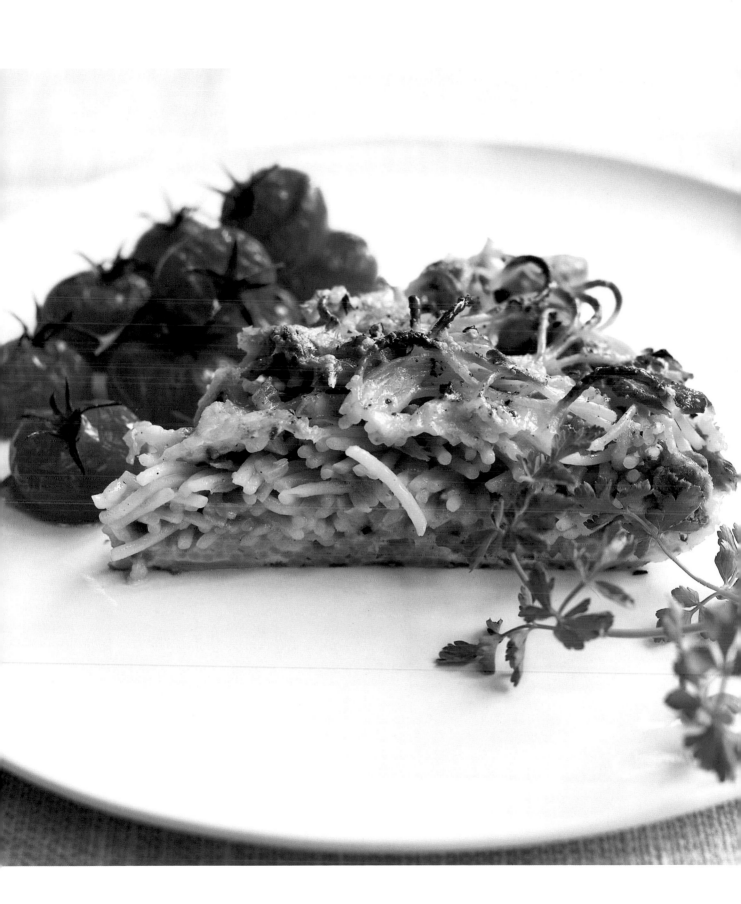

lemon and haddock penne bake

Here, juicy flakes of smoked haddock, penne, and broccoli are baked in a creamy lemon sauce beneath a crisp cheese and crumb topping. This dish is a great way to enjoy broccoli, an excellent source of vitamin C and antioxidants that may help to reduce the risk of certain cancers.

SERVES 4

11 oz penne or other pasta shapes
1 lb skinless smoked haddock (finnan haddie)
  fillet
2 cups lowfat milk
2 tablespoons butter
1 tablespoon all-purpose flour
grated zest and juice of 1/2 lemon
2 1/2 cups broccoli florets, blanched
1/3 cup grated sharp Cheddar cheese
1/3 cup fresh white bread crumbs
freshly ground black pepper

1 Preheat the oven to 400°F. Cook the pasta in a large pan of boiling water according to the package directions, until *al dente* (cooked but still a bit firm to the bite).

2 Place the smoked haddock in a shallow pan, pour in the milk, and cover with a circle of parchment paper. Bring to a simmer and poach gently for 3–4 minutes. Remove the smoked haddock to a plate, reserving the milk.

3 Melt the butter in a small pan, stir in the flour, and cook over a gentle heat for 2 minutes. Slowly whisk in the reserved milk and cook for 5 minutes. Add the lemon zest and juice, and season the sauce with pepper to taste.

4 Drain the pasta as soon as it is cooked. Roughly flake the haddock and mix with the pasta and broccoli florets. Place in a large gratin or baking dish and pour the sauce over.

5 Mix together the Cheddar cheese and bread crumbs, then scatter over the top. Bake for 10 minutes or until bubbling hot and golden. Serve immediately, accompanied by a tomato salad.

Boston baked beans, sausage, and macaroni

Now that you can buy so many different types of canned beans, soaking and slow-cooking dried beans is becoming a thing of the past. Make sure you use good-quality sausages for this dish, as they'll be less fatty and will have more flavor. Finish with shavings of sharp Cheddar and peppery arugula leaves—the stronger the cheese, the less you need to provide flavor.

SERVES 4

6 oz macaroni
4 good-quality fresh pork sausages
2 cups tomato purée
3 tablespoons light brown sugar
3 tablespoons tomato ketchup
3 tablespoons white wine vinegar
dash of Worcestershire sauce
14 oz canned pinto beans, drained and rinsed
14 oz canned cannellini beans, drained and
  rinsed
large handful of arugula leaves
1¹/₂ oz sharp Cheddar cheese, in shavings
freshly ground black pepper

1 Preheat the oven to 400°F. Cook the sausages in a nonstick frying pan for 12–15 minutes, turning frequently, until browned and cooked through.

2 Meanwhile, cook the macaroni in a large pan of boiling water according to the package directions, until *al dente* (cooked but still a bit firm to the bite).

3 Combine the tomato purée, sugar, tomato ketchup, wine vinegar, and Worcestershire sauce in a saucepan. Stir together, then add the pinto and cannellini beans, and simmer for 10 minutes.

4 Drain the macaroni and add to the beans. Cut each sausage into 4 chunky pieces and stir into the bean mixture, then season to taste. Spoon into a baking dish and bake for 8–10 minutes until piping hot. Just before serving, scatter the arugula leaves and cheese shavings over the top.

simply dressed pasta

Endlessly versatile, pasta is a great staple and carrier of flavors, and it is not fattening—unless, of course, you dress it to be so. It is essentially an energy food, high in beneficial complex carbohydrate, low in fat, and a useful source of protein. Dried pasta is often considered superior to that bought fresh; if made from 100 percent durum wheat, it is slightly higher in protein. There is an extraordinary range of shapes, sizes, and colors to choose from.

For perfect results, cook your pasta in the largest pan of boiling water you can provide, without a lid. Use the time given on the package as a guide, but keep testing toward the end of cooking. The pasta is ready when it's "*al dente*," or "firm to the tooth"—not hard and chalky, and not soggy. Stop the cooking by tipping a cup of cold water into the pan, then drain quickly, leaving a little water on the pasta. Try these great ideas for pasta. Each serves 4.

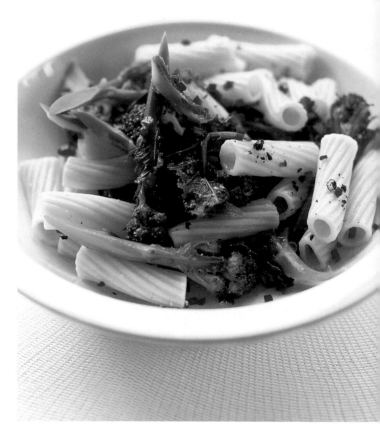

chilied broccoli rabe

Cook 12 oz rigatoni in boiling water until al dente. Trim 12 oz broccoli rabe, separate the stems, and steam for 4 minutes or until *al dente*. Drain the cooked pasta and toss with the broccoli, 2 seeded and minced hot red chili peppers, a squeeze of lemon juice, and 2 tbsp extra virgin olive oil. Grind lots of black pepper over the top and serve.

roasted tomato and olive sauce

Put 8 oz each cherry tomatoes and baby plum tomatoes into a roasting pan. Add 1 cup each sliced black and green olives, a pinch of sugar, 2 tbsp olive oil, and plenty of black pepper. Roast at 400°F for 20–25 minutes. Meanwhile, cook 12 oz tagliatelle in a large pan of boiling water until *al dente*. Drain well and toss with the roasted tomato and olive sauce, mixing in all the juices.

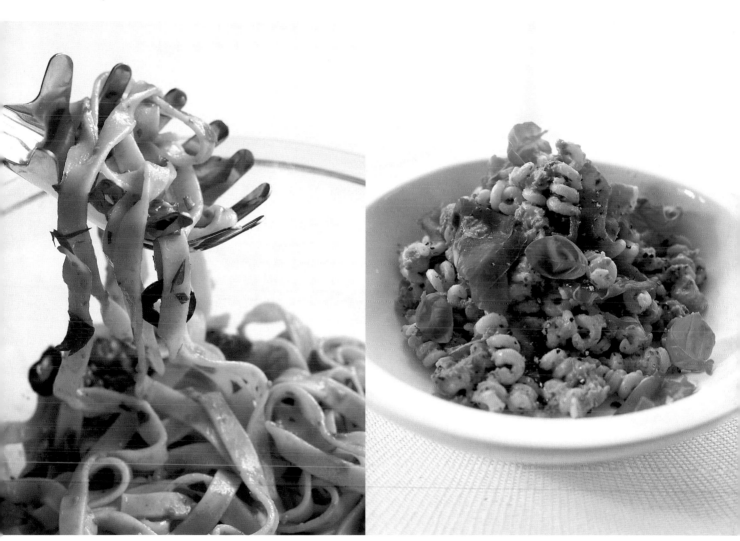

Moroccan-dressed chick peas

Heat 2 tsp olive oil in a pan, stir in 1 thinly sliced red onion, and steam-fry for 5 minutes. Stir in 2 tbsp harissa paste, 6 tbsp white wine, and 14 oz canned crushed tomatoes. Simmer gently for 10 minutes. Add 14 oz canned chick peas (garbanzo beans), drained, and heat through. Season to taste. Meanwhile, cook 12 oz penne in plenty of boiling water until *al dente*. Drain the pasta and return to the pan. Toss with the chick pea sauce and serve.

pea pesto with ricotta and prosciutto

Cook 12 oz pasta spirals in boiling water until *al dente*. Cook 1½ cups frozen green peas in boiling water for 3 minutes, then drain, reserving ½ cup liquid. In a food processor, whiz the peas with 5 tbsp basil leaves, ½ cup ricotta cheese, 2 tsp lemon juice, 1 crushed garlic clove, and the reserved liquid until fairly smooth; add pepper to taste. Gently heat the pea pesto. Drain the pasta and toss with the pesto. Serve topped with wafer-thin slices of prosciutto and basil leaves.

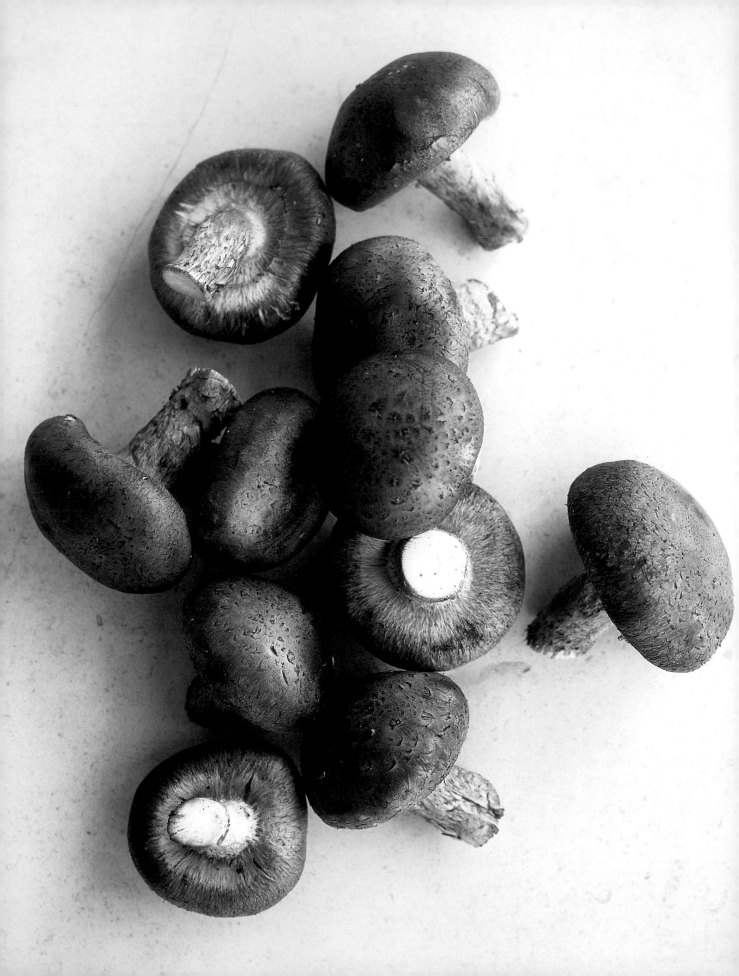

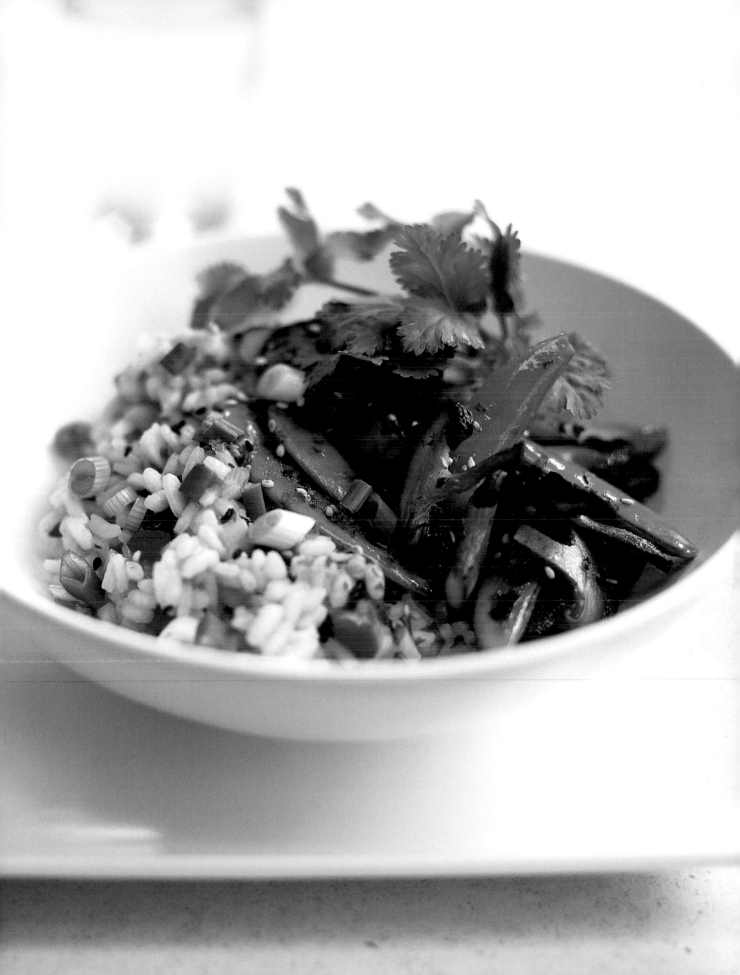

Japanese rice with sugarsnaps and shiitake mushrooms

This sticky risotto, infused with Japanese flavors, is a tasty lowfat alternative to a traditional Italian risotto. Furikake seasoning, which is made from nutritious black and white sesame seeds and seaweed, has a delicious nutty flavor. You buy furikake in a jar—look for it in Asian markets and wholefood stores. *Illustrated on page 139*

SERVES 4

2 sachets instant miso soup powder
1 tablespoon olive oil
2-inch piece fresh ginger, peeled and minced
1 garlic clove, peeled and crushed
1 hot red chili pepper, seeded and minced
½ bunch of green onions, trimmed and chopped
1 cup arborio rice
12 oz sugarsnap peas, trimmed
9 oz shiitake mushrooms, sliced
2 tablespoons furikake (Japanese seasoning)
2 teaspoons mirin
freshly ground black pepper
cilantro sprigs for garnish

1 Mix the miso powder with 4 cups boiling water in a saucepan and keep at a gentle simmer on a low heat.

2 Heat ½ tablespoon olive oil in a pan over a medium heat, add the ginger, garlic, chili pepper, and green onions, and cook for 1 minute. Stir in the rice.

3 Keeping the rice over a medium heat, add the miso, a ladleful at a time, stirring constantly and making sure each addition is absorbed before adding more (this will take approximately 20 minutes). The rice is cooked when it looks thick and creamy, but still retains a little firmness. Season to taste.

4 Heat the remaining oil in a nonstick wok or large nonstick frying pan. Add the sugarsnap peas and mushrooms, and stir-fry for 2–3 minutes. Stir in the furikake seasoning and mirin, and cook for a further 30 seconds.

5 Spoon the rice into warm serving bowls, and add the stir-fried sugarsnaps and mushrooms. Garnish with cilantro sprigs and serve immediately.

green rice soubise

Wholegrain brown rice contains more fiber than white rice, but it does take longer to cook. Fortunately, this wholegrain rice dish is baked, so once it's in the oven you can forget about it. Onions are one of the richest sources of flavonoids—antioxidants that help our immune system. This simple dish is finished with a scattering of creamy ricotta, a versatile lowfat cheese.

SERVES 4

1 tablespoon olive oil
2 onions, peeled and minced
2 garlic cloves, peeled and crushed
2 cups short-grain brown rice, rinsed
1 lemon, cut into 4 wedges
5 cups vegetable stock
2¹/₂ cups broccoli florets
1¹/₄ cups frozen green peas, thawed
1 bunch of green onions, trimmed and
  chopped
¹/₂ cup ricotta cheese
2 tablespoons torn basil
freshly ground black pepper

1 Preheat the oven to 400°F. Heat the oil in a large, shallow stovetop-to-oven casserole, add the onions, and cook over a medium heat for 5 minutes, stirring occasionally. Add the garlic and cook for a further 2 minutes until the onions are softened and golden.

2 Add the rice and lemon wedges, and stir well. Pour in the stock and bring to a boil. Cover with foil, transfer to the oven, and bake for 45–50 minutes. In the meantime, blanch the broccoli in boiling water for 2–3 minutes, then drain and refresh under cold water.

3 Remove the rice dish from oven and stir in the broccoli, peas, and green onions. Season well and crumble the ricotta on top. Bake, uncovered, for a further 6–8 minutes or until the rice is tender and most of the liquid has been absorbed. Scatter the basil over and serve.

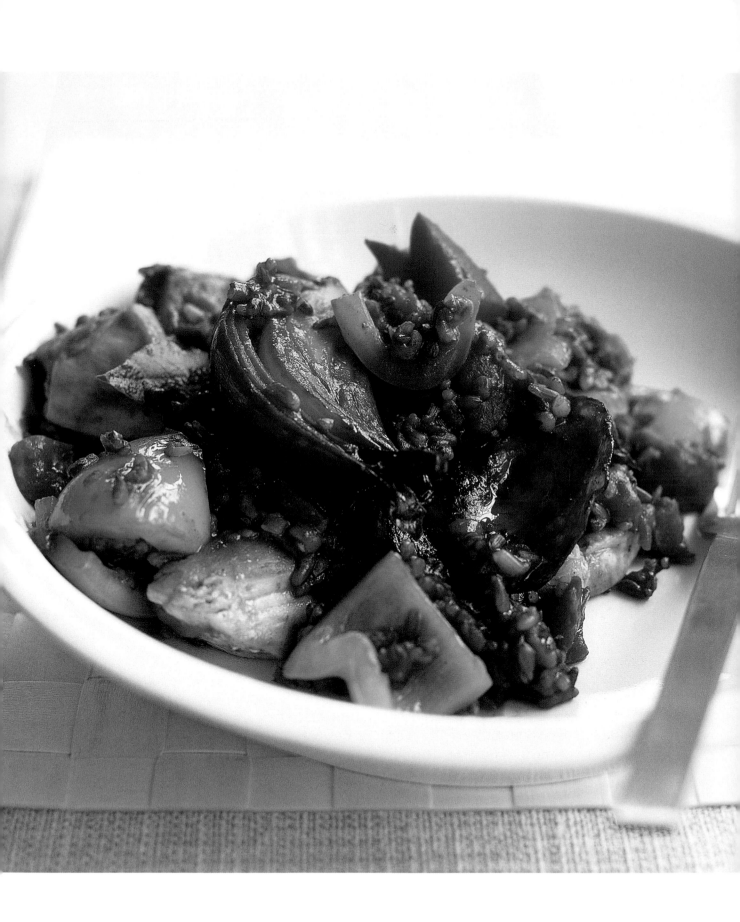

jambalaya

Red rice has a good flavor, nutty texture (due to the fact that the bran has been left on the rice grains), and a distinctive color. To make this jambalaya, I have cooked the rice separately to speed things up, and I've flavored the dish with pimenton, a smoked sweet paprika. Bell peppers are a good source of beta-carotene, the plant form of vitamin A, which may help to reduce the risk of some forms of cancer and heart disease.

SERVES 4

2 boneless, skinless chicken breast halves, each about 5 oz
1 each red, yellow, and orange bell peppers
2 cups long-grain red rice
3 oz smoked chorizo sausage, sliced
1 tablespoon olive oil
1 red onion, peeled and cut into 8 wedges

2 garlic cloves, peeled and crushed
1½ teaspoons smoked paprika
pinch of ground cloves
3 bay leaves
14 oz canned crushed tomatoes
1 cup vegetable stock
freshly ground black pepper

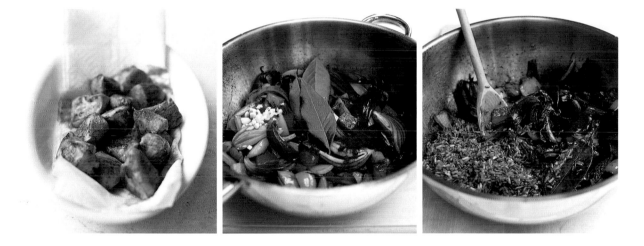

1 Cut the chicken into 1-inch pieces. Halve, core, and seed the bell peppers, then chop roughly. Cook the rice in a pan of boiling water according to the package directions.

2 Meanwhile, heat a large shallow pan, add the chorizo slices, and cook for 30 seconds on each side until golden. Remove with a slotted spoon and set aside. Add the chicken to the pan and sauté for 10 minutes until golden all over. Remove from the pan and drain on paper towels.

3 Add the olive oil to the pan. Add the red onion and bell peppers, and cook for 5 minutes or until the vegetables are lightly golden. Stir in the garlic, smoked paprika, cloves, and bay leaves. Cook for 1 minute.

4 Stir in the drained, cooked rice, chorizo, and chicken. Add the tomatoes and stock, and bring to a boil. Simmer for 8–10 minutes or until most of the liquid has been absorbed. Season to taste and serve.

baked chicken and thyme risotto

This oven risotto doesn't require constant stirring, but the result is still creamy in texture. It is rich in protein and starchy carbohydrates. Dried porcini mushrooms lend a superb, intense flavor that combines well with the garlic and thyme.

SERVES 4

1 oz dried porcini mushrooms
4 skinless, boneless chicken thighs
2 garlic cloves, peeled and crushed
2 teaspoons thyme leaves, plus extra for garnish
1 tablespoon olive oil
1 large onion, peeled and minced
4 cups vegetable stock
1¹/₂ cups arborio rice
¹/₂ cup white wine
freshly ground black pepper

1 Put the dried mushrooms in a bowl, pour in 1 cup warm water, and let soak for 30 minutes. Preheat the oven to 375°F.

2 With a small sharp knife, slash the chicken thighs on the diagonal, just cutting through the flesh. Rub them all over with the garlic and thyme, then season with pepper.

3 Heat the oil in a large, shallow stovetop-to-oven casserole and cook the chicken for 2–3 minutes each side until golden. Remove from the pan and set aside.

4 Add the onion to the pan with a splash of stock and cook gently for 5 minutes or until softened. Add the rice and stir for 1 minute. Add the drained mushrooms and cook for a further minute. Pour in the wine and cook for 2 minutes until it has evaporated.

5 Add the rest of the stock and bring to a boil. Season well. Place the chicken thighs on top of the rice. Cover with a lid and transfer to the oven to bake for 20–25 minutes until the rice is just cooked and all the stock has been absorbed. Scatter extra thyme leaves on top, then serve.

crab and salmon kedgeree

This modern version of a traditional Anglo-Indian breakfast dish is surprisingly spiced with Thai green curry paste. Crab tastes delicious in the spicy rice, while roasted salmon strips provide an attractive topping. A cooling carrot and cilantro raita is the ideal accompaniment.

SERVES 4
2 teaspoons olive oil
1 onion, peeled and minced
2 tablespoons green Thai curry paste
2 tablespoons mango chutney
$2/3$ cup white wine
$1^{1}/_{4}$ cups vegetable stock
2 cups basmati rice, rinsed
12 oz skinless salmon fillet
6 oz canned white crabmeat, drained
FOR THE RAITA:
1 cup plain yogurt
1 small carrot, peeled and grated
$1/4$ cup chopped cilantro
freshly ground black pepper

1 Preheat the oven to 400°F. Heat the oil in a pan, stir in the onion, and steam-fry for 10 minutes or until soft and golden. Stir in the Thai curry paste and mango chutney, and cook for 1 minute. Pour in the wine and stock, then cook until reduced to about 1 cup.

2 Meanwhile, cook the rice according to the package directions. Cut the salmon into 8 strips lengthwise and place on a nonstick baking sheet. Roast for 5–7 minutes until just cooked.

3 Mix all the ingredients for the raita together in a bowl and season well with black pepper.

4 Drain the rice and gently toss with the reduced curry paste mixture, then fold in the crabmeat. Spoon the kedgeree onto warm serving plates, top with the salmon strips, and serve immediately, with the carrot and cilantro raita.

salads and vegetables

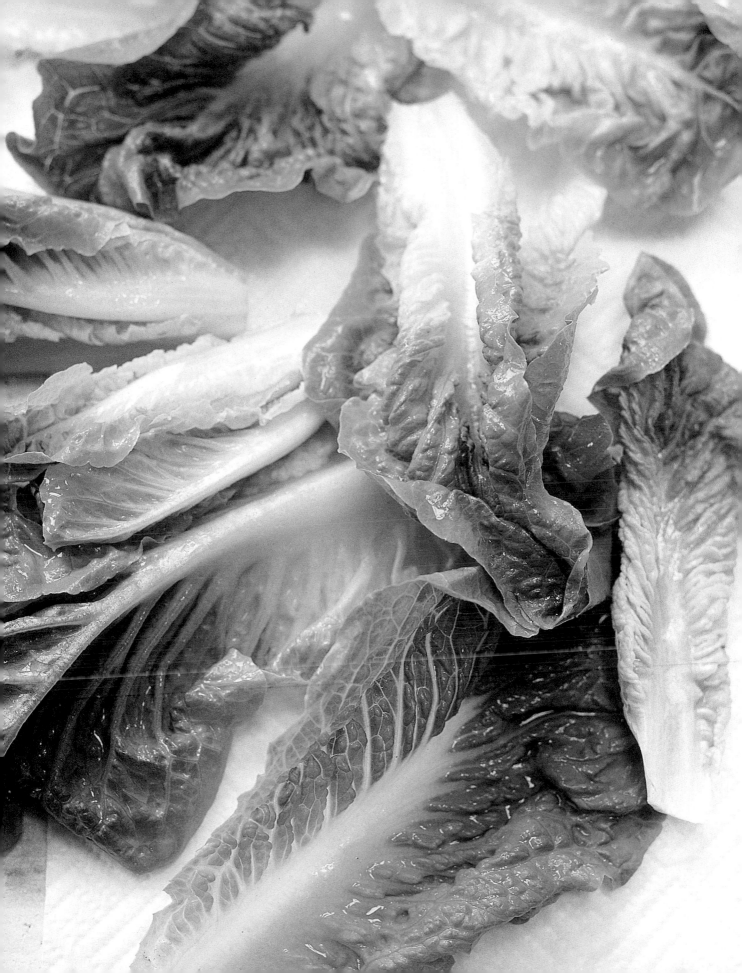

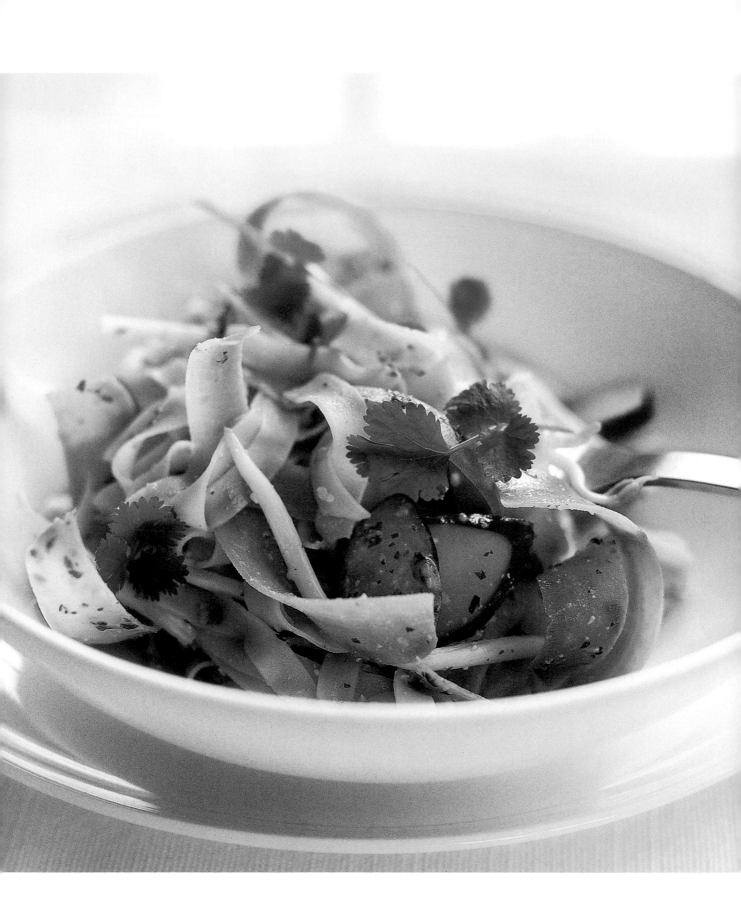

cashew and rice noodle salad

Rice noodles are great for anyone on a wheat-free diet and they're so quick to cook. Toast the cashew nuts to give maximum flavor to the dressing, keeping an eye on them because they can quickly scorch and acquire a bitter taste. Cashew nuts contain protein, minerals—especially magnesium—and some B vitamins. Carrot ribbons are an attractive addition; cucumber and zucchini ribbons look good in salads, too.

SERVES 4

$1/3$ cup cashew nuts
2 medium carrots, peeled
2 tablespoons light soy sauce
juice of 1 large orange
3 garlic cloves, peeled and crushed
2 tablespoons grapeseed oil
$1/2$ cup cilantro leaves
9 oz rice noodles, cooked
1 bunch of radishes, trimmed and sliced
1 heaped cup bean sprouts
freshly ground black pepper

1 Place the cashew nuts in a small frying pan over a medium heat and toast for about 3 minutes, shaking the pan constantly, until an even golden color. Set aside to cool slightly.

2 Using a swivel vegetable peeler, pare along the length of the carrots to make long, thin ribbons. Set aside.

3 Set aside a handful of cilantro leaves. Place the rest in a food processor with the toasted cashew nuts, soy sauce, orange juice, garlic, and grapeseed oil. Whiz until fairly smooth, then season to taste.

4 Toss the noodles, carrot ribbons, radishes, and bean sprouts together. Pour the dressing over and toss well to coat evenly. scatter over the reserved cilantro to serve.

harissa beefsteak tomatoes with tabbouleh

Tabbouleh is a fragrant Middle Eastern salad made with nutty bulghur wheat, lemon juice, olive oil, and lots of freshly chopped mint and parsley. Here, it is served with roasted tomatoes that are spiked with harissa paste. Pine nuts, high in essential fatty acids, give this dish some added protein, making it a complete meal for vegetarians.

SERVES 4

1¹/₂ cups bulghur wheat

4 beefsteak tomatoes, halved

2 tablespoons harissa paste

2 tablespoons extra virgin olive oil, plus extra
   for drizzling

juice of 1 lemon

¹/₄ cup chopped mint

¹/₄ cup chopped Italian parsley

¹/₂ cup pine nuts, toasted

freshly ground black pepper

plain yogurt for serving

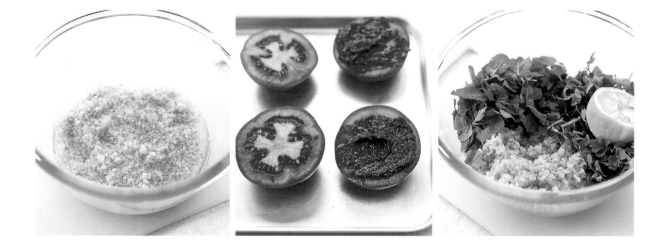

1 Preheat the oven to 425°F. Put the bulghur wheat in a bowl and cover with cold water. Let soak for 30 minutes. Drain if necessary.

2 Place the tomatoes, cut-side up, on a nonstick baking sheet and spread with the harissa paste. Roast for 10–12 minutes or until just softened but still holding their shape.

3 Meanwhile, toss the bulghur wheat with the olive oil, lemon juice, and chopped mint and parsley. Season to taste.

4 Spoon the tabbouleh onto four plates and top each serving with two roasted tomato halves. Scatter the toasted pine nuts on top and drizzle a little extra olive oil over. Serve with yogurt.

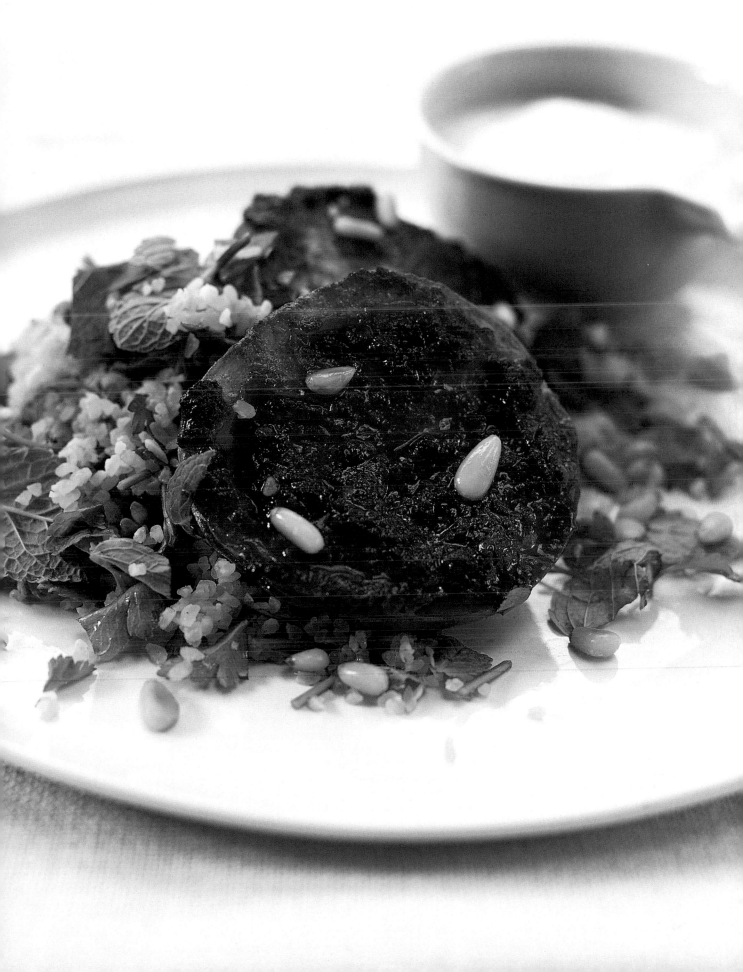

guacamole and bean salad on toasted pita

Chunky guacamole, made from nutrient-rich avocados, partners a Mexican-style bean and watercress salad that's rich in fiber and iron. Toasted pita bread is the ideal foil.

SERVES 4

2 ripe avocados

juice of 1 lime

2 shallots, peeled and minced

10 cherry tomatoes, quartered

1 hot red chili pepper, seeded and minced

2 garlic cloves, peeled and crushed

2 tablespoons extra virgin olive oil

14 oz canned red kidney beans, drained

1 bunch of watercress, tough stems removed

6 pita breads, toasted

freshly ground black pepper

1   Halve, pit, and peel the avocados, then cut into ½-inch cubes. Place in a bowl and sprinkle with the lime juice. Add the shallots, tomatoes, chili pepper, 1 garlic clove, and 1 tablespoon olive oil, and gently mix together. Season with black pepper.

2   Toss the kidney beans with the remaining garlic and oil, then toss in the watercress and season well. Spoon onto toasted pita breads and top with the chunky guacamole.

warm peppered goat cheese salad

Goat cheese has a tangy, gutsy flavor, so a little goes a long way. Here, it is coated in black pepper, then pan-grilled until golden and served on salad leaves with an unusual red bell pepper and lentil dressing.

SERVES 4

2 goat cheeses with rind, each 3½ oz

1 tablespoon freshly ground black pepper

2 tablespoons cooked lentils

1 small red bell pepper, seeded and minced

3 tablespoons extra virgin olive oil

juice of ½ lemon

4 handfuls of baby salad leaves

1   Cut each cheese in half horizontally and coat all over with the pepper, pressing to adhere. Heat a nonstick grill pan until hot. Add the peppered cheese, cut-side down, and cook for 2 minutes or until colored and crusty. Turn over and cook for a further 1 minute or until the cheese is soft but still retaining its shape.

2   Meanwhile, mix together the lentils, red bell pepper, olive oil, and lemon juice in a small bowl; season well. Arrange the salad leaves on serving plates, top with the pan-grilled goat cheese, and spoon the dressing over the top.

warm potato and egg salad

This is a lovely fresh combination of colorful ingredients. Tossing the baby new potatoes in the mustard dressing while they are still hot encourages them to soak up all the flavors. Potatoes are a useful source of vitamin C, potassium, and fiber. The salad is topped with soft-boiled eggs and sprinkled with garden cress—one of my favorite salad items.

SERVES 4

1½ lb baby new potatoes, scrubbed

8 oz green beans, trimmed and halved

9 oz cherry tomatoes, halved

4 eggs

1 small bunch of garden cress or watercress, trimmed

FOR THE DRESSING:

2 teaspoons Dijon mustard

1 tablespoon white wine vinegar

1 shallot, peeled and minced

1 garlic clove, peeled and crushed

3 tablespoons extra virgin olive oil

freshly ground black pepper

1 Place the baby potatoes in a pan of cold water, bring to a boil, and simmer for 20 minutes or until just tender.

2 Meanwhile, make the dressing. Whisk the Dijon mustard, wine vinegar, shallot, garlic, and olive oil together in a bowl and season to taste.

3 Drain the potatoes and toss them in the dressing. Set aside to cool for 5 minutes. Blanch the green beans in boiling water for 1 minute, then drain and refresh in cold water; drain well. Add the beans and tomatoes to the potatoes and toss to mix.

4 Meanwhile, put the eggs in a pan with enough boiling water to cover and boil gently for 2 minutes. Put the eggs under running cold water, then remove and very carefully peel them.

5 To serve, spoon the salad into bowls, top each serving with a soft-boiled egg, and scatter the cress over. Serve immediately.

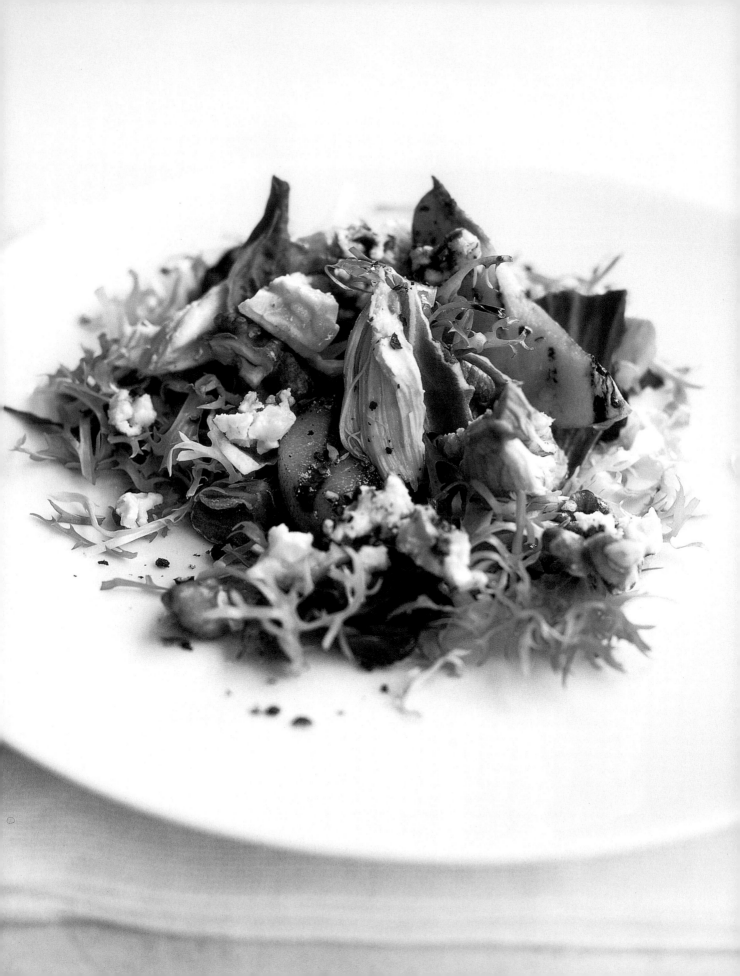

pan-grilled pear, chicken, and endive salad

Here, sweet pears complement bitter salad leaves, tangy Roquefort, and cooked chicken to delicious effect. Toasted walnuts provide a crunchy contrast and enrich the nutrient value—they are rich in essential fatty acids and a useful source of protein, B vitamins, vitamin E, and minerals. Chicken is an excellent, lowfat protein food.

SERVES 4

2 large, ripe Bartlett or Comice pears
4 handfuls of mixed curly endive and radicchio
10 oz cooked chicken breast meat
1/2 cup walnuts, toasted
1/3 cup crumbled Roquefort cheese

FOR THE DRESSING:
2 tablespoons extra virgin olive oil
2 tablespoons balsamic vinegar
freshly ground black pepper

1 Halve, quarter, and core the pears, then cut into thick slices. Heat a nonstick grill pan until very hot. Add the pear slices and grill for 1 minute on each side or until lightly charred. Remove and set aside.

2 For the dressing, whisk the olive oil and balsamic vinegar together in a small bowl. Season with pepper to taste.

3 Tear the chicken into bite-sized pieces. Arrange the salad leaves on four serving plates and top with the chicken, pears, toasted walnuts, and crumbled blue cheese. Drizzle the dressing over the salad and grind a little extra black pepper on top. Serve with bread.

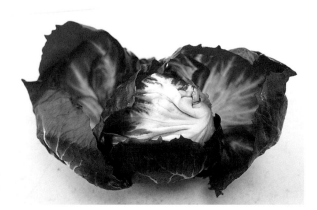

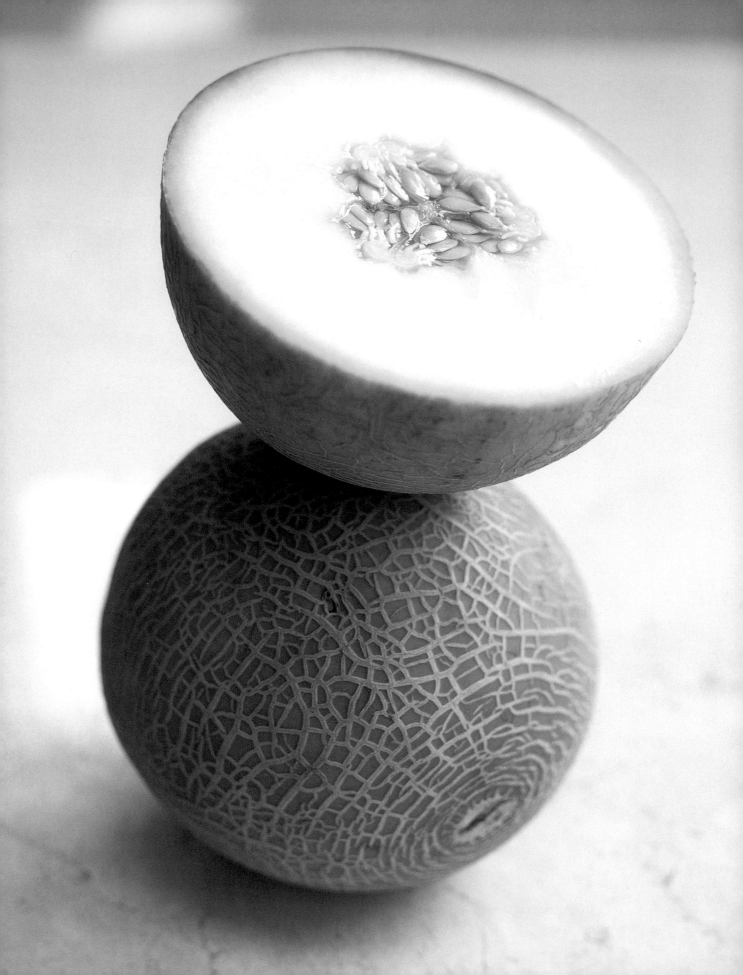

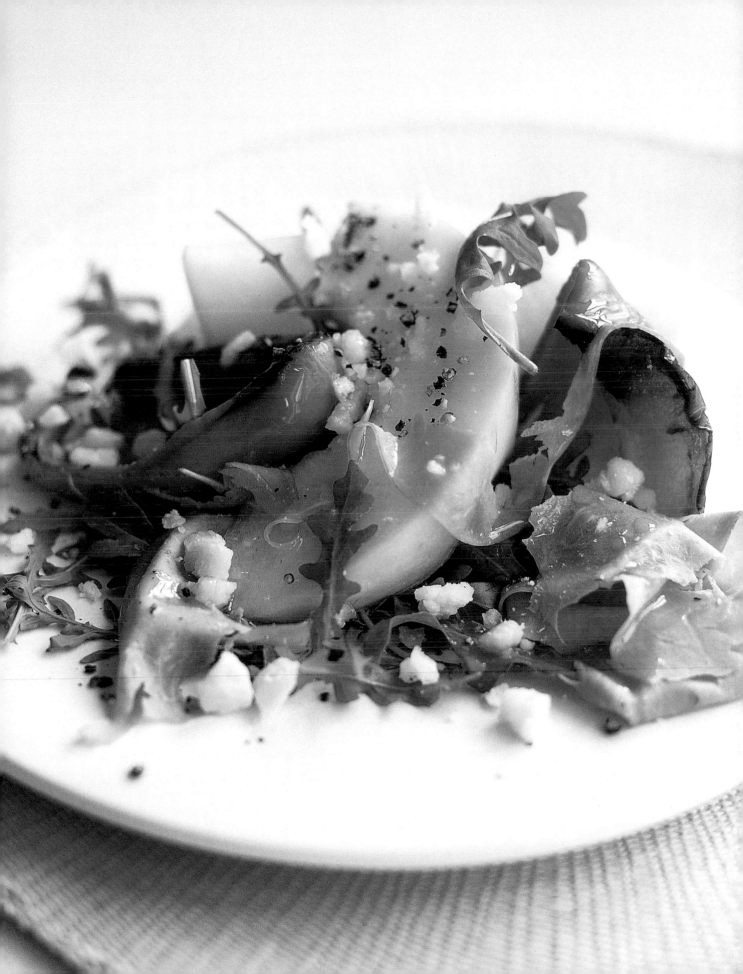

melon with sweet ham

This is a colorful summer salad of ripe, juicy melon and roasted orange bell peppers topped with honey-roast ham, tangy pecorino cheese, and arugula. Pecorino, an Italian sheep's milk cheese, is rich in protein and calcium. *Illustrated on page 157*

SERVES 4

3 large orange bell peppers

2 teaspoons olive oil

1 ripe cantaloupe melon

4 handfuls of arugula leaves

4 oz wafer-thin honey-roast ham slices

1/3 cup crumbled pecorino cheese

freshly ground black pepper

a little extra virgin olive oil for drizzling

1 Preheat the oven to 425°F. Quarter, core, and seed the bell peppers, then place in a roasting pan and drizzle the olive oil over them. Roast for 20–25 minutes. Set aside to cool.

2 Cut the melon in half and scoop out the seeds. Cut each half into four wedges. Arrange the arugula on serving plates and top with the melon, roasted peppers, and ham. Scatter the cheese over the top, and finish with a generous grinding of black pepper and a drizzle of olive oil.

mango-crab salad

Fragrant mango, fresh crab, crisp salad leaves, and a spicy mayonnaise make a healthy salad with a difference. Mango is a rich in vitamins C, A, and E. Like all shellfish, crab is a good source of protein, B vitamins, and some minerals, including zinc.

SERVES 4

1 head romaine lettuce, trimmed

1 hothouse cucumber

1 small, ripe mango

4 cups fresh white crabmeat

1 lime, cut into wedges

FOR THE DRESSING:

3 tablespoons reduced-fat mayonnaise

6 tablespoons plain yogurt

2 tablespoons hot (spicy) mango chutney

large squeeze of lime juice

1 Tear the romaine leaves into pieces. Peel, halve, and seed the cucumber, then slice on the diagonal. Peel, halve, and slice the mango away from the central seed. Arrange these ingredients on a large platter or individual plates.

2 Top with the crabmeat. Mix the dressing ingredients together in a bowl. Serve the crab salad with the dressing, lime wedges, and some good whole-wheat bread.

spinach and Parmesan polenta bake

I've called this a polenta bake because it has an Italian accent—the cornmeal is flavored with nutrient-rich spinach, Parmesan, and nutmeg. Folding in beaten egg whites gives it a lovely puffy finish. This is delicious served with a simple plum tomato salad.

SERVES 4

2 teaspoons olive oil

1 onion, peeled and minced

1$^2/_3$ cups lowfat milk

1 cup yellow cornmeal

3 extra large eggs, separated

$^1/_2$ cup grated Parmesan cheese

1 teaspoon grated nutmeg

1$^1/_2$ cups roughly chopped baby spinach leaves

freshly ground black pepper

FOR THE SALAD:

6 ripe plum tomatoes

splash of balsamic vinegar

bunch of basil leaves

1   Preheat the oven to 400°F. Lightly oil a 5-cup baking dish.

2   Heat the olive oil in a pan, add the onion, and gently cook for 10 minutes or until softened and golden brown. Pour in the milk and 1$^1/_4$ cups water, and bring to a boil.

3   Rain in the cornmeal, stirring well until smooth, then remove from heat. Beat in the egg yolks, Parmesan, nutmeg, and spinach, and season generously.

4   Beat the egg whites until they form soft peaks, then gently fold into the cornmeal mixture. Spoon into the prepared dish. Bake for 20–25 minutes or until slightly puffed up and golden brown.

5   Meanwhile, thinly slice the plum tomatoes and arrange on a serving plate. Drizzle the balsamic vinegar over the tomatoes, scatter with the basil, and add a grinding of pepper. Serve with the polenta bake.

potatoes

Cooked with a new attitude, potatoes have a role in a healthy diet. They're rich in complex carbohydrate and contain useful amounts of fiber, Vitamin C, and protein. Some nutrients are concentrated just under the skin, so scrub potatoes rather than peel them if possible.

For crisp-skinned, fluffy baked potatoes, use russets, also called Idaho potatoes. Bake for about 1 hour in a hot oven, turning halfway—don't be tempted to use the microwave. Russets are also good for perfect creamy mash: cut into pieces and boil for 15–20 minutes until tender, then drain and mash with a little hot milk or plain yogurt and black pepper. For extra taste, add grain mustard or horseradish. Boiling potatoes and new potatoes, both of which have waxy flesh, are ideal for salads: boil for 15–20 minutes and dress with reduced-fat mayonnaise and chopped herbs. Or, toss them in a little olive oil and roast until crisp. Each of the potato recipes here serves 4.

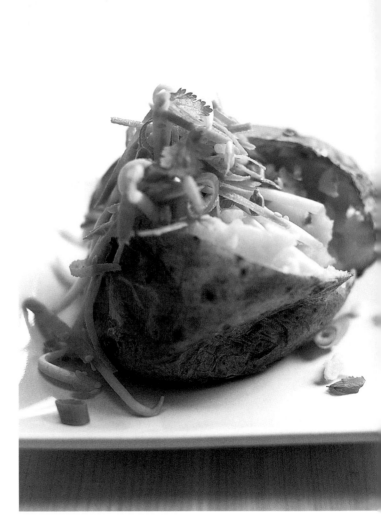

baked potatoes with sesame and sunflower slaw
Bake 4 large potatoes at 400°F for about 1 hour until tender, turning them over halfway through cooking. Meanwhile, mix together 1 tbsp soy sauce, 2 tbsp sour cream, 1 tbsp reduced-fat mayonnaise, and 3 tbsp each of toasted sunflower and sesame seeds. Toss this dressing with 3 peeled and grated carrots, 1½ cups beansprouts, and 4 chopped green onions. Split open the hot baked potatoes, pile in the slaw, and top with cilantro leaves.

potato and onion cakes

Scrub 3 medium potatoes, grate, and dry well on paper towels. Mix with 1 finely sliced red onion, 2 tbsp olive oil, a little nutmeg, and black pepper. Divide into 4 portions and press into thin cakes on a preheated nonstick baking sheet. Bake at 400°F for 25–30 minutes or until golden. Serve on a salad of baby spinach leaves and crumbled, crisp-fried, lean bacon with a drizzle of balsamic vinegar.

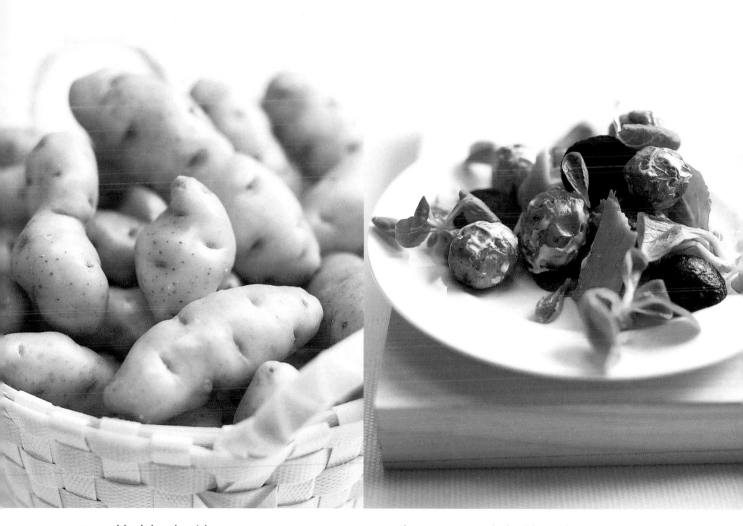

potato and leek broth with pesto greens

Heat ½ tbsp olive oil in a large pan. Add 2 chopped leeks, 1 peeled and chopped large sweet potato, 2 peeled and chopped white potatoes, and a bay leaf. Cover and cook for 10 minutes. Pour in 3½ cups vegetable stock and a splash of white wine. Simmer for 15–20 minutes. Meanwhile, cook 3 cups shredded Savoy cabbage with 2 tbsp water in a covered wok for 2 minutes; stir in 1 tbsp pesto sauce. Ladle the broth into bowls and top with the cabbage.

roasted new potato salad with smoked trout

Toss 2 lb baby new potatoes with black pepper and 1 tbsp olive oil. Roast at 375°F for 45 minutes or until tender. Mix together 2 tsp grain mustard, 1 tsp Dijon mustard, 4 tbsp plain yogurt, the juice of ½ lemon, 1 tbsp water, and ¼ tsp honey. Divide 2 large handfuls of corn salad (mâche), 9 oz halved, cooked baby beets, 1 cup flaked smoked trout, and the hot potatoes among 4 plates and drizzle the dressing over the top.

vegetable hash with eggs

A mixed root vegetable hash of potatoes, carrots, and leeks topped with protein-rich eggs makes an appetizing, healthy lunch or supper. Always buy eggs from cage-free or free-range hens if you can. For best results, use a good-quality nonstick pan to fry the hash.

SERVES 4

1 lb russet or all-purpose potatoes, peeled
2 tablespoons olive oil
2 leeks, trimmed and finely shredded
2 carrots, peeled and grated
4 medium or large eggs
1 tablespoon chopped Italian parsley
freshly ground black pepper

1 Grate the potatoes, then squeeze out as much liquid as possible with your hands and dry on paper towels. Preheat the broiler.

2   Heat the oil in a 9- to 10-inch nonstick frying pan (suitable for use under the broiler). Add the leeks and cook, stirring, for 2 minutes. Stir in the grated potatoes and carrots, then lightly spread out the mixture in the pan. Fry over a medium heat for 10 minutes until golden underneath.

3 Place the pan under the broiler and cook for 5 minutes or until the hash is golden on top. Remove from the broiler and make four indentations in the surface of the hash.

4 Break the eggs into the indentations, grind a little black pepper over, and scatter the chopped parsley on top. Cover with a lid or baking sheet, place back over a medium heat, and cook for 4–5 minutes or until the eggs are cooked to your taste. Serve hot.

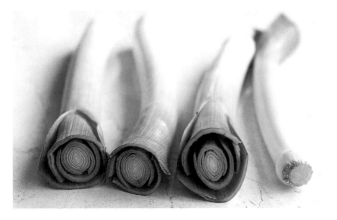

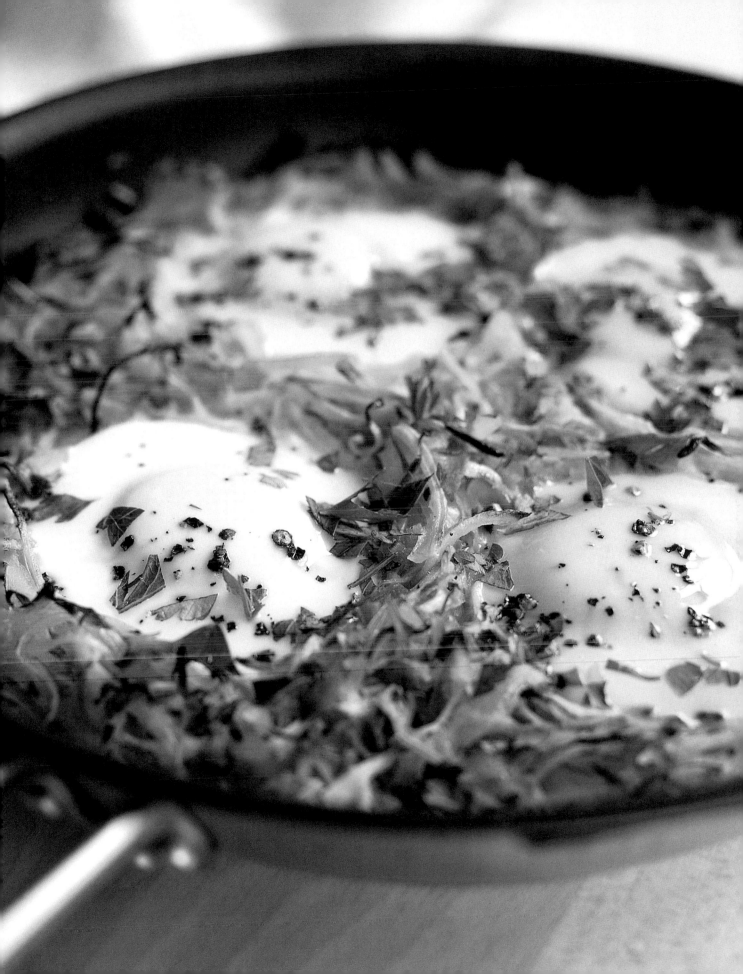

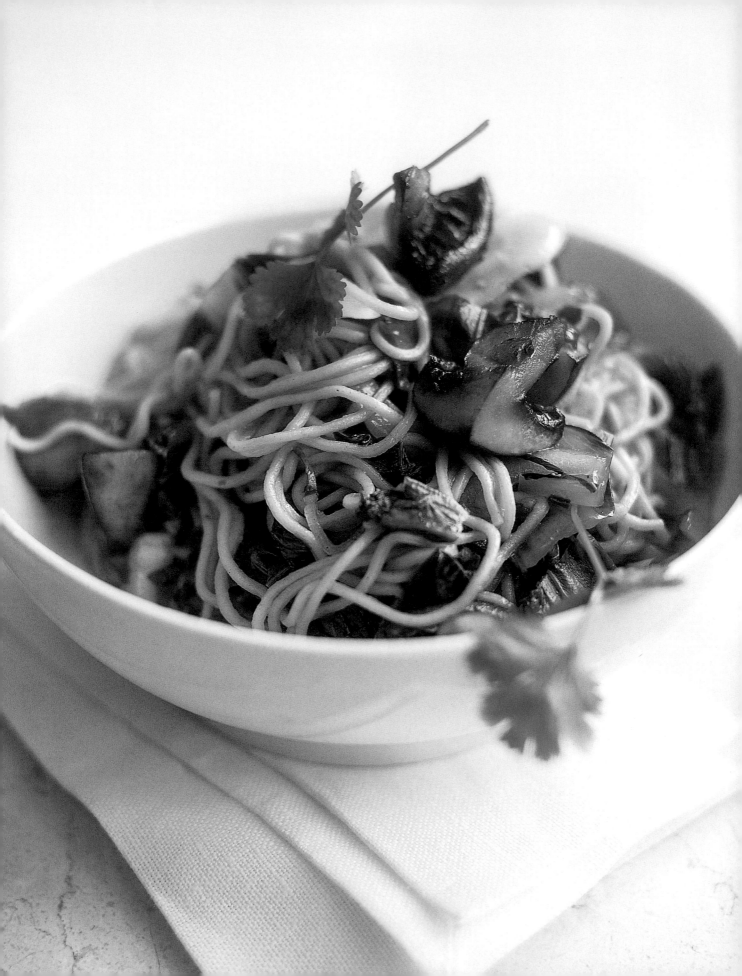

bok choy and noodle stir-fry

Bok choy is particularly delicious in stir-fries, although you could substitute other Chinese cabbage, Napa cabbage, or even Savoy cabbage, if you prefer. Stir-frying is one of the healthiest ways of cooking these leafy green vegetables, because it helps to preserve their vitamin C content—C is the least stable of all vitamins. Don't wash mushrooms: simply wipe them clean with paper towels.

SERVES 4

9 oz thin egg noodles
2 tablespoons peanut oil
8 oz crimini mushrooms, halved or
  quartered if large
2 garlic cloves, peeled and crushed
2 hot red chili peppers, seeded and minced
3 small heads bok choy, shredded
2 tablespoons soy sauce
2 tablespoons sweet chili dipping sauce
freshly ground black pepper
cilantro sprigs, for garnish

1 Cook the egg noodles in boiling water according to the package directions.

2 At the same time, prepare the stir-fry. Heat the peanut oil in a nonstick wok or large nonstick frying pan. Add the mushrooms and garlic, and stir-fry for 1–2 minutes. Stir in the chili peppers and cook for 30 seconds. Add the bok choy and stir-fry for 1 minute.

3 Toss in the drained egg noodles and the soy and chili sauces, and season with pepper to taste. Heat through for 1 minute or until the noodles are piping hot. Divide among warm bowls, garnish with cilantro, and serve at once.

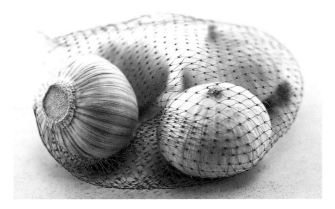

roasted Mediterranean vegetable tart

This impressive upside-down tart is very easy to make, using a bread mix. Roasted eggplant, zucchini, red bell peppers, red onion, and cherry tomatoes are baked under the dough, then it's all turned over and topped with crumbled feta to serve. Feta cheese is a sheep's milk cheese—useful for anyone with an intolerance to cow's milk protein.

SERVES 6

1 eggplant

2 zucchini, trimmed

2 red bell peppers, halved and seeded

1 red onion, peeled

1 cup cherry tomatoes

2 tablespoons olive oil

1/2 lb package bread mix

1/3 cup chopped black olives

1 cup crumbled feta cheese

2 tablespoons torn basil leaves

freshly ground black pepper

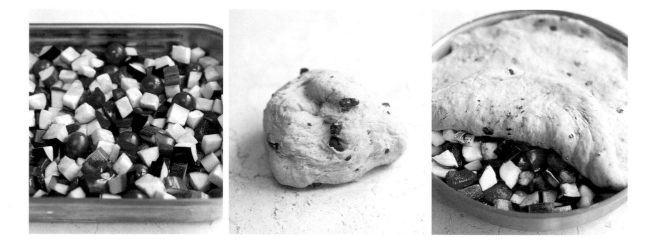

1 Preheat the oven to 425°F. Chop the eggplant, zucchini, bell peppers, and onion into 1/2-inch chunks. Place in a roasting pan with the cherry tomatoes, in a single layer. Drizzle the olive oil over, season well with black pepper, and roast for 25–30 minutes.

2 Meanwhile, make up the bread dough following the package directions, adding the chopped black olives as you knead the dough. Set aside.

3 Transfer the roasted vegetables to a shallow, round, nonstick baking pan or dish that is about 9 inches in diameter. Roll out the olive dough to a round a little larger than the pan and place on top of the vegetables. Press the dough down well and to the rim of the pan. Bake for 15–20 minutes.

4 Cool for a few minutes, then place an inverted large serving plate over the pan, turn them over together, and lift off the pan. Tap the pan to make sure all the vegetables come away. Scatter the feta and basil over the vegetables and cut into wedges to serve.

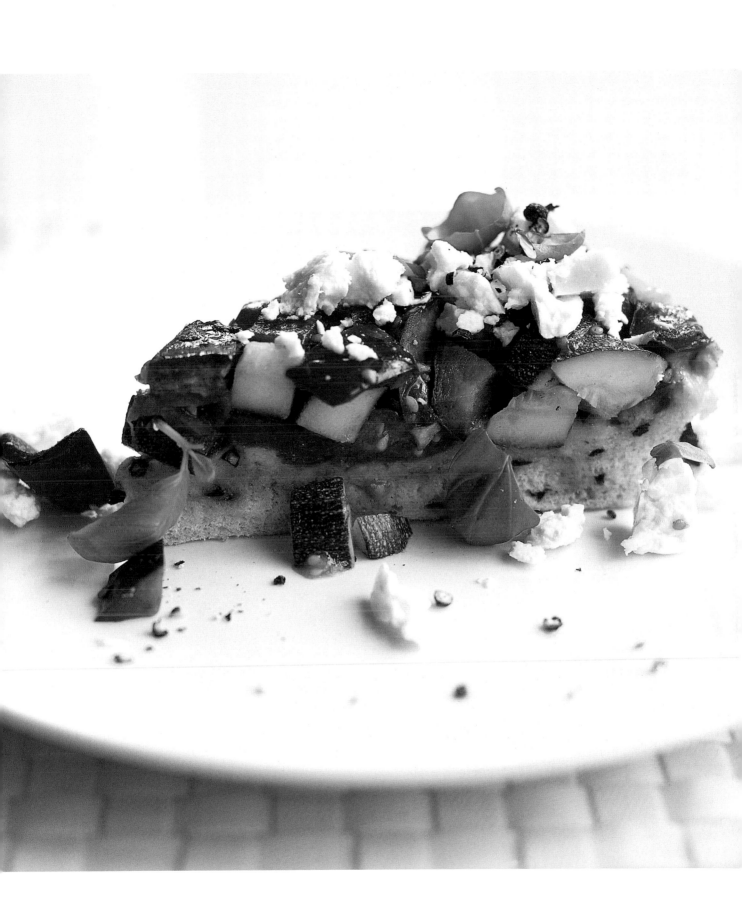

butternut barley risi

Barley, an interesting grain with a nutty texture, is very under-rated grain in my opinion. It is easily digested and highly nutritious, providing a good source of fiber, calcium, and protein. It works perfectly in this cross between a rich stew and a risotto, which is topped with roasted chunks of butternut squash to serve.

SERVES 4

1/2 cup pearl barley, rinsed
1 large butternut squash, peeled and seeded
2 tablespoons olive oil
1 large leek, trimmed and finely sliced
1 garlic clove, peeled and minced
2 bay leaves
2 large strips of orange peel
5 cups vegetable stock
4 tablespoons chopped Italian parsley
freshly ground black pepper
freshly grated Parmesan cheese for serving

1 Soak the pearl barley in cold water to cover for 30 minutes. Preheat the oven to 400°F.

2 Cut the butternut squash into 1-inch pieces. Place in a large roasting pan, drizzle 1 tablespoon of the olive oil over them, and season with black pepper. Roast for 35–40 minutes until tender and slightly caramelized.

3 Meanwhile, heat the remaining oil in a large saucepan. Add the leek and garlic, and steam-fry for 5 minutes until softened. Drain the pearl barley and add to the leek, along with the bay leaves, orange peel, and stock. Bring to a boil, then simmer gently for 30 minutes or until the barley is just tender.

4 Stir the parsley into the risi and season with black pepper. Ladle into warm bowls and top with the roasted butternut squash and Parmesan to serve.

sweet vegetable and coconut green curry

This speedy vegetable curry has a wonderful creamy texture, as coconut milk is used as the stock. Tofu, or soybean curd, is an important source of high-quality protein, especially for vegetarians. Tofu also contains beneficial antioxidants, calcium, and other essential minerals, plus B vitamins and vitamin E. Peas are a must in the freezer, as they are such a useful standby and provide vitamin C, which helps the body to absorb iron.

SERVES 4

2 teaspoons olive oil

1 onion, peeled and minced

2^1/$_2$ tablespoons Thai green curry paste

3 medium sweet potatoes, peeled

14 oz canned coconut milk (preferably reduced-fat)

1 cinnamon stick

5 oz marinated tofu

1^1/$_2$ cups frozen green peas

2 tablespoons chopped cilantro leaves

1 Heat the olive oil in a pan. Add the onion and steam-fry for 5 minutes, then stir in the curry paste and cook for 1 minute.

2 Meanwhile, cut the sweet potatoes into 1-inch chunks. Add to the spiced onion and stir to coat with the mixture. Pour in the coconut milk and ^{2}/$_3$ cup water, and add the cinnamon stick. Bring to a boil, then cover and simmer for 20 minutes.

3 Stir in the tofu and peas, and cook for 3 more minutes. Scatter the cilantro over the top and serve with Thai fragrant rice.

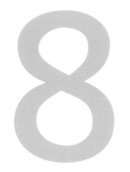 desserts

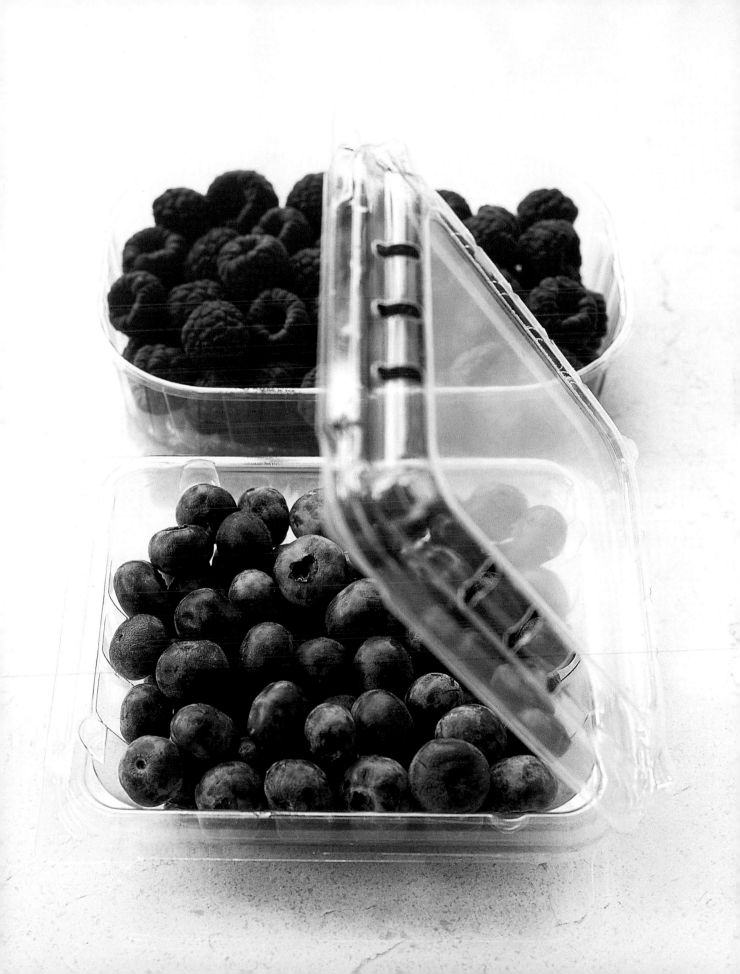

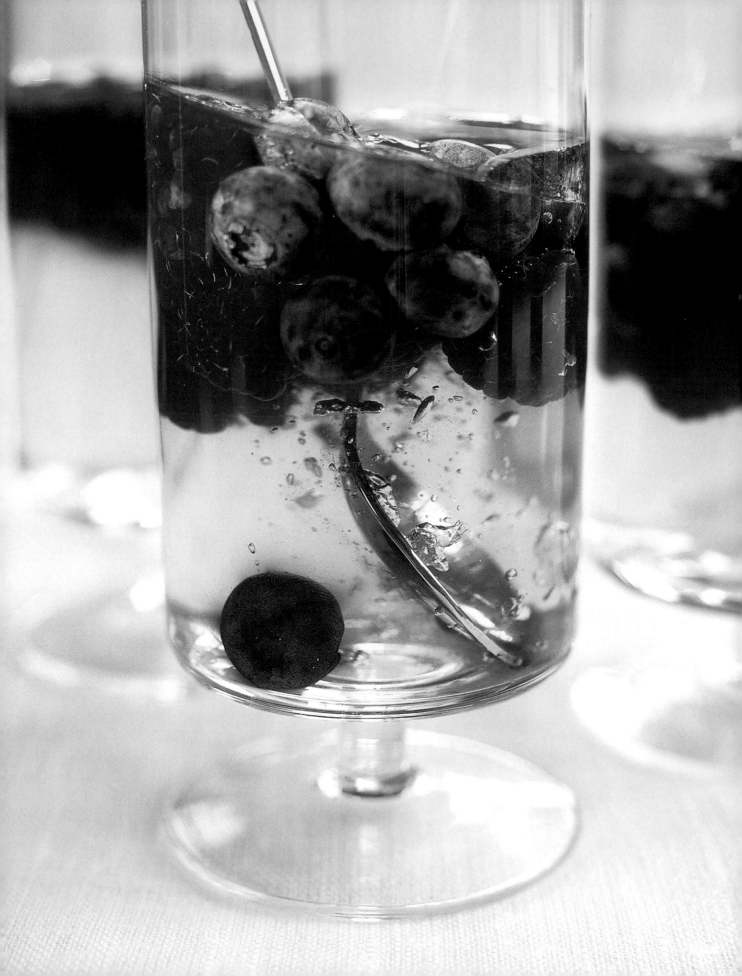

lime and berry gelatins

This refreshing lime dessert, flavored with raspberries and blueberries, is a delightful way of adding to your five-a-day fruit and veggies. Raspberries are a rich source of vitamin C, which helps the body to absorb iron and also helps improve the health of your skin. If preferred, you can substitute vegetarian gelatin and use according to the package directions, but note that this product may not achieve such a crystal clear set.

SERVES 4

5 tablespoons sweetened lime juice concentrate,
  plus extra for drizzling
1 envelope unflavored gelatin
1 cup raspberries
1 cup blueberries

1   Dilute the lime juice concentrate with 2 cups cold water. Pour 4 tablespoons into a small pan, sprinkle the gelatin on top, and set aside for 10 minutes.

2   Divide the raspberries and blueberries among four wine glasses or goblets.

3   Place the pan containing the softened gelatin over a very gentle heat and swirl in the pan until the gelatin has completely dissolved; do not overheat. Gradually pour in the remaining lime liquid, stirring well over a low heat.

4   Pour the liquid into the glasses, then chill for 3 hours or until set. Just before serving, spoon a little extra lime juice concentrate on top.

meringue parfaits with pineapple and orange salad

Crushed meringue and toasted hazelnuts are folded into creamy plain yogurt, a good source of calcium. The mixture is semi-frozen in ramekins, then unmolded and served with a zingy, vitamin C-rich pineapple and orange salad.

SERVES 4

2 cups thick plain yogurt (preferably nonfat Greek-style yogurt, if available)
4 baked meringue shells, crumbled
1/2 cup chopped hazelnuts, toasted

FOR THE FRUIT SALAD:

1 small pineapple
3 large oranges

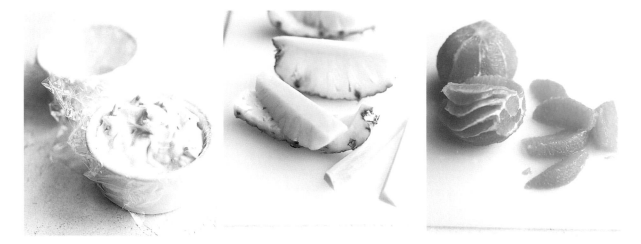

1 Line four 5-oz ramekins with plastic wrap. Put the yogurt in a large bowl and gently fold in the meringues and chopped hazelnuts. Spoon the mixture into the prepared ramekins and freeze for 2½ hours or until semi-frozen.

2 With a sharp knife, cut away the skin from the pineapple, then cut into wedges and remove the core. Cut each wedge into thin slices lengthwise.

3 Using a small sharp knife, peel the oranges, removing all the white pith, then cut out the segments from between the membranes. Gently toss the pineapple slices and orange segments together in a serving bowl.

4 Unmold the semi-frozen parfaits onto serving plates and remove the plastic wrap. Scatter some extra toasted chopped hazelnuts on top, if desired, and arrange a few pieces of the fruit alongside. Serve accompanied by the rest of the pineapple and orange salad.

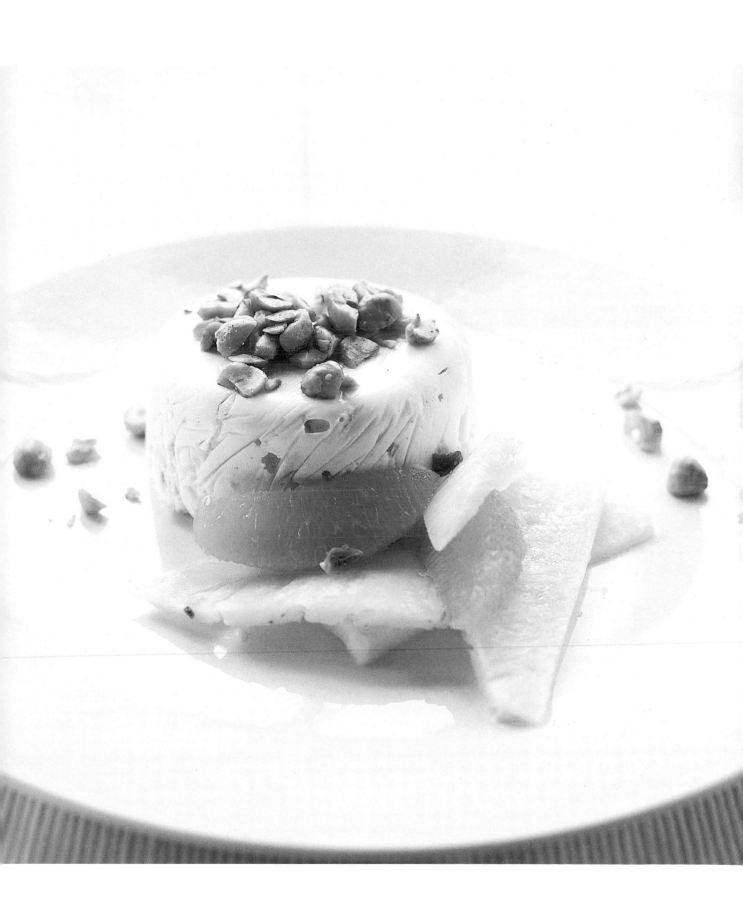

apples and pears

Juicy, succulent, versatile, and often under-rated, apples and pears feature in most fruit bowls. They make delectable desserts as well as great high-energy snacks.

There are numerous varieties of apples available. Most can be eaten raw and used in cooking. Popular varieties include refreshing and crisp Pippins and Granny Smiths, sweet-tart Lady Apples and Braeburn, and sweet Galas and Fujis. For baked apples that keep their shape, choose Rome Beautys or Gravensteins.

Pears at their peak of ripeness have a sublime, delicate flavor. Most varieties can be eaten raw as well as cooked; choose firm pears if you are going to cook them. Bartletts and Comice are the ultimate dessert pears, and are superb for juicing. Boscs hold their shape well when baked or poached. And don't forget pears canned in natural juice, which are a useful standby. Each of these apple or pear recipes serves 4.

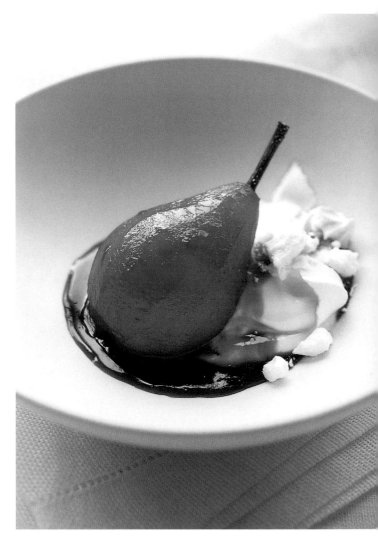

red berry-pear soup

Peel 4 ripe pears, retaining the stems. Put 1¼ cups cranberry juice, 1 cup apple juice, pared rind and juice of ½ orange, 4 cloves, 1 cinnamon stick, 1 rosemary sprig, and ¼ cup sugar in a wide saucepan. Heat gently to dissolve the sugar, then add the pears. Bring to a boil, then cover with parchment paper, reduce the heat, and poach for 30–40 minutes until tender. Serve warm or cold, with light sour cream and some crumbled baked meringue.

apple marmalade with thick cinnamon toasts

Place 4 chopped large tart-sweet apples in a pan with 1 cup sliced dried apricots, the grated zest and juice of 2 large oranges, and 2 tbsp dark brown sugar. Cook over a medium heat for 12–15 minutes until the apples are soft and jamlike. Split and toast 4 cinnamon bagels and serve with the warm apple marmalade.

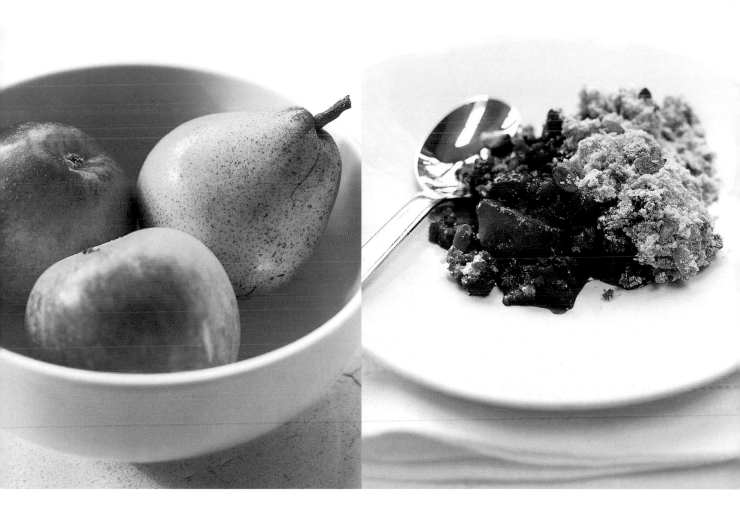

pears with mocha fondue

Pour ⅔ cup lowfat milk into a pan and add 4 oz (4 squares) chopped bittersweet chocolate. Place over a medium heat and stir until melted. Dissolve 1 tsp instant coffee in 1 tbsp boiling water. Stir into the chocolate mixture and simmer for 2 minutes. Serve the mocha sauce in small espresso cups or teacups with ripe pear wedges for dipping.

apple and blackberry crisp

Place 6 peeled and chopped large tart-sweet apples and 2 cups blackberries in a shallow baking dish. For the topping, rub 2 tbsp diced butter into 1¼ cups all-purpose flour until the mix resembles crumbs. Stir in ¼ cup light brown sugar, 2 tbsp pumpkin seeds 2 tbsp sunflower seeds, and 2 tbsp orange juice. Scatter the topping over the fruit with a little extra sugar. Bake at 400°F for 35–40 minutes.

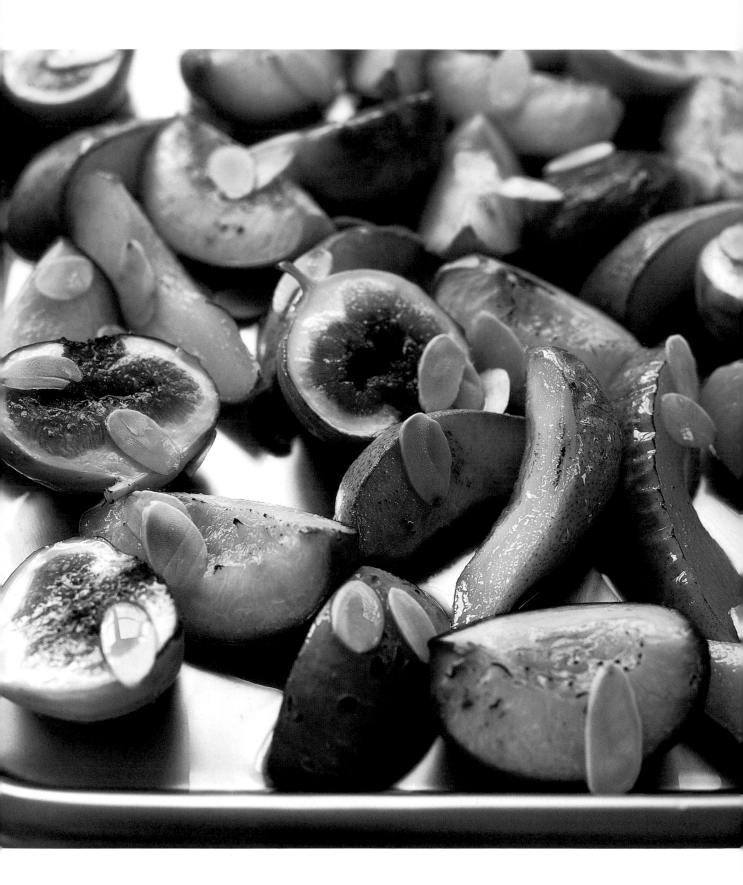

roasted maple fruits

Here's an interesting way to increase your daily fruit intake: nectarines, fresh figs, and pears roasted in maple syrup and wine. I like to serve them hot, with vanilla frozen yogurt.

SERVES 4

3 small nectarines, halved and pitted
3 ripe pears, peeled, quartered, and cored
3 tablespoons maple syrup
3 tablespoons white wine or apple juice
4 fresh figs, halved
1/2 cup sliced almonds

1   Preheat the oven to 400°F. Cut the nectarines and pears into thick wedges and place in a small roasting pan.

2   Pour the maple syrup and wine or apple juice over the fruits and toss well to coat evenly. Roast for 10 minutes.

3   Add the figs to the roasting pan and baste with the pan juices. Scatter the sliced almonds over the fruits, then roast for a further 12–15 minutes until the fruit is glazed and the nuts are golden. Serve hot, with frozen yogurt or light sour cream.

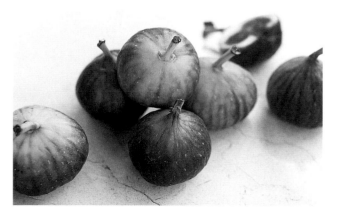

chocolate and prune mousse

Prunes are the secret ingredient in this lowfat mousse. Like other dried fruits, they are highly nutritious and naturally sweet, which means you can reduce the amount of sugar required in the recipe. Prunes are a good source of potassium, magnesium, iron, and fiber, and contain antioxidants that may help to protect the body from disease.

SERVES 4–6

4 oz (4 squares) bittersweet chocolate
1 cup pitted prunes
2 tablespoons brandy (optional)

3 egg whites
1 tablespoon superfine sugar
unsweetened cocoa powder, for dusting

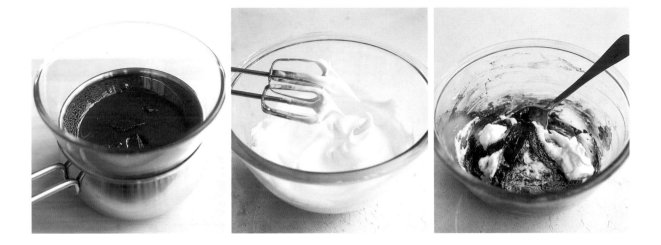

1 Break up the chocolate and place in a heatproof bowl set over a pan of hot water. Leave until melted, then stir until smooth and set aside to cool slightly.

2 Place the prunes in a saucepan and pour in ⅔ cup water. Simmer very gently, stirring occasionally, until very, very soft. Transfer the warm prunes and any remaining liquid to a blender or food processor, and add the brandy if using. Whiz to a smooth purée.

3 Beat the egg whites in a large, clean bowl until stiff, then whisk in half of the sugar. Add the remaining sugar and beat until thick and glossy.

4 Stir the melted chocolate into the prune purée and beat together. Stir in a spoonful of the beaten egg whites to loosen the mixture, then carefully fold in the remaining egg whites.

5 Spoon the mousse into small espresso coffee cups or glasses and chill until required. Just before serving, dust with cocoa powder.

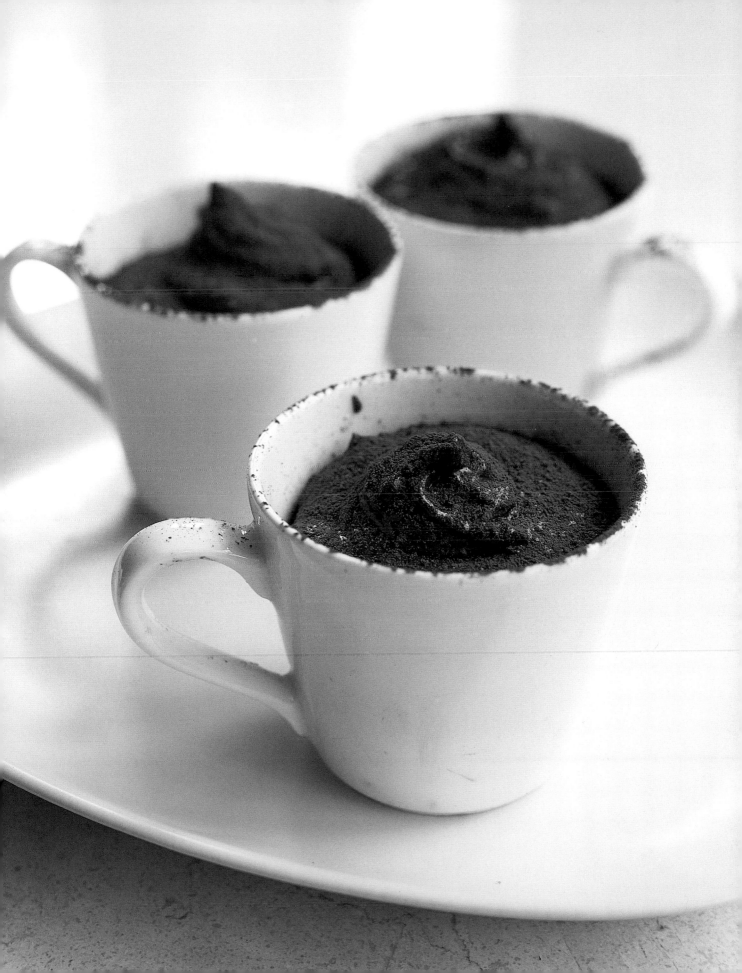

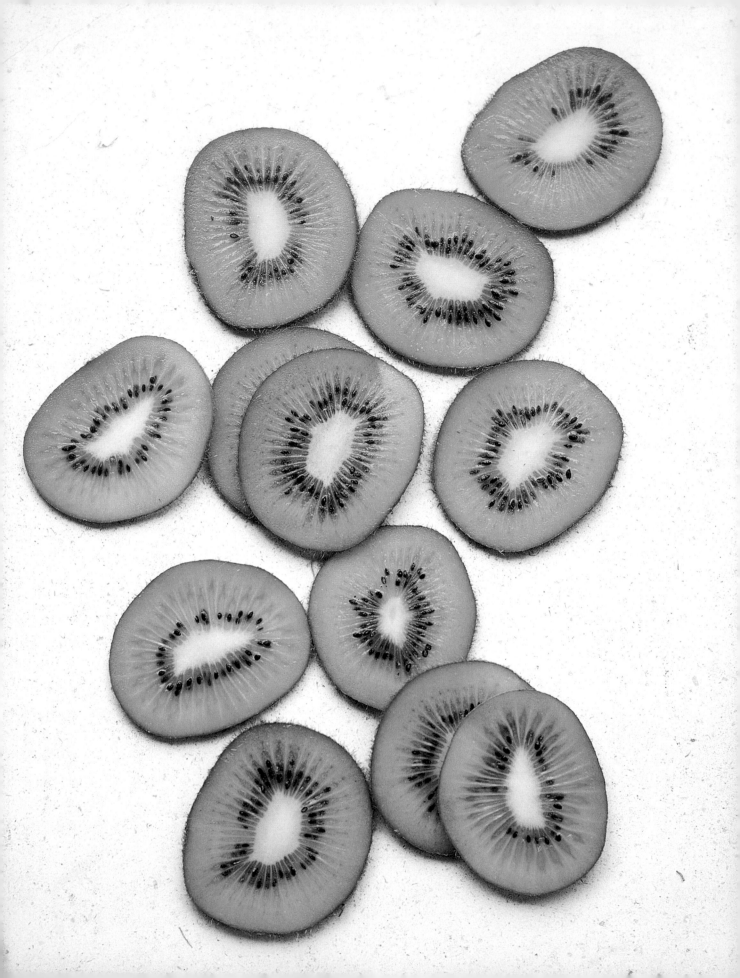

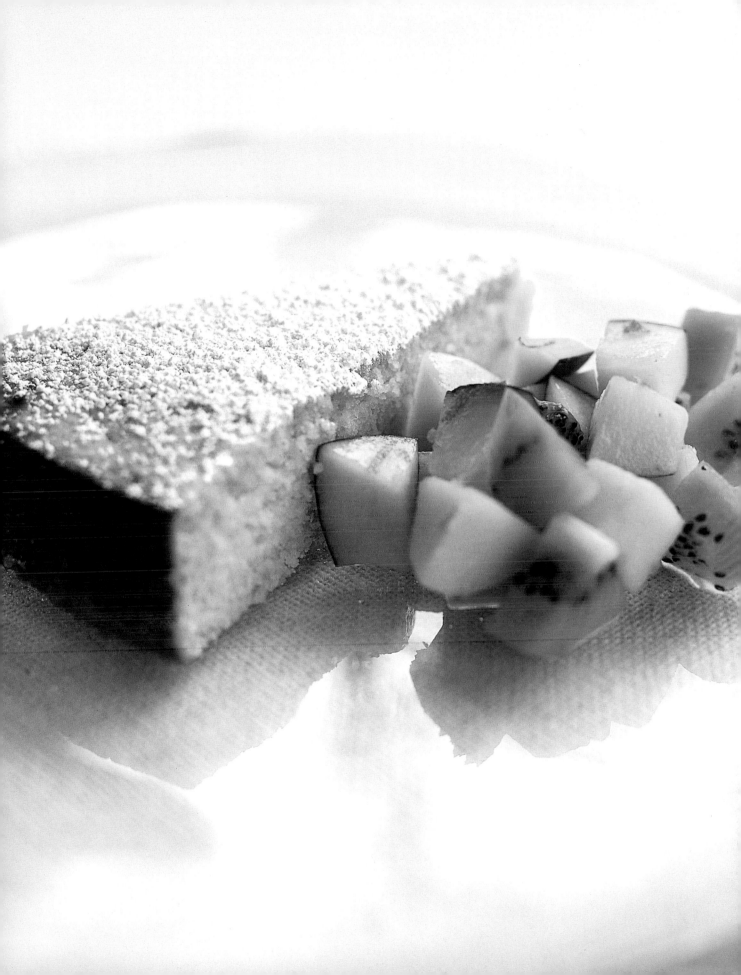

citrus almond cake with tropical fruit salsa

A cooked orange (skin and all) is puréed and incorporated into this cake batter, to create a deliciously moist cake, without any butter. To serve, simply dust with confectioners' sugar and accompany with a refreshing, vitamin C-rich, tropical fruit salsa. *Illustrated on page 183*

SERVES 4

1 large orange, washed and quartered

3 eggs, beaten

$1/2$ cup ground almonds

$2/3$ cup yellow cornmeal

$1/2$ teaspoon baking powder

$2/3$ cup granulated sugar

grated zest and juice of 1 lemon

confectioners' sugar, for dusting

FOR THE FRUIT SALSA:

2 kiwi fruit, peeled

1 small, ripe mango, peeled and cut away from
   the central seed

1 nectarine, halved and pitted

grated zest and juice of $1/2$ lime

1 Place the orange in a saucepan, add enough water to cover, and bring to a boil. Lower the heat and simmer for 25–30 minutes.

2 Preheat the oven to 375°F. Lightly grease and flour an 8-inch round cake pan.

3 Remove the orange from the pan and chop roughly, discarding the seeds. Put the warm chopped orange into a food processor and blend until very smooth. Add the eggs, ground almonds, cornmeal, baking powder, granulated sugar, and lemon zest, and whiz briefly to combine.

4 Pour the cake batter into the prepared pan and bake for 25–30 minutes until just firm. Let cool in the pan slightly, then, using a fork, prick the top of the cake all over. Spoon the lemon juice over it.

5 For the fruit salsa, chop the fruits and toss together, along with the lime zest and juice. Dust the cake with confectioners' sugar and serve cut into wedges, with the fruit salsa.

fruit salad platter with biscotti

This is a stylish, fun way of enjoying more than one of your five-a-day fruit and veggies. Packed with vitamin C and sprinkled with a satisfying crunch of biscotti, this dessert couldn't be easier. As an alternative, you can crumble brandy snaps over the fruit. Strawberries are an exceptional source of vitamin C and high in pectin, which is a soluble fiber that helps reduce cholesterol levels in the body. They also have strong antioxidant properties.

SERVES 4

1 small, ripe melon
1 large, ripe mango
2 large kiwi fruit, peeled
2 ripe nectarines, halved and pitted
8 oz strawberries
juice of 1 orange
4 oz biscotti

1　Halve the melon and scoop out the seeds with a spoon, then cut away the rind. Thickly slice the melon flesh. Peel the mango and cut into chunks, slicing the flesh away from the central seed. Quarter the kiwi fruit and nectarines.

2　Arrange all of the fruits attractively on a large platter. Cover with plastic wrap and chill until ready to serve. Place the biscotti in a plastic bag and lightly crush with a rolling pin.

3　Just before serving, squeeze the orange juice over the chilled fruits. Scatter the crushed biscotti on top and serve at once.

hot plum-muffin pudding

Bubbling hot, fresh plums nestle beneath a cinnamon-scented topping in this "comfort food" pudding that is surprisingly low in fat and high in fiber. It resembles a cobbler, except that the topping is more like a muffin batter than a biscuit dough. Other fruit, such as apricots, peaches, and nectarines, can be substituted for the plums.

SERVES 4

1¼ lb plums, halved and pitted

finely grated zest and juice of 1 orange

2 tablespoons light brown sugar, plus extra
  for sprinkling

1 cup all-purpose flour

2 teaspoons baking powder

½ teaspoon ground cinnamon

3 tablespoons granulated sugar

3 tablespoons milk

3 tablespoons plain yogurt

1 egg

1 tablespoon butter, melted

1   Preheat the oven to 350°F. Place the plums in a shallow oven-to-table dish in a single layer. Drizzle the orange juice over the fruit and sprinkle with the brown sugar. Bake for 15 minutes.

2   Meanwhile, sift the flour, baking powder, and cinnamon into a bowl and stir in the granulated sugar. Make a well in the center.

3   In another bowl, whisk together the milk, yogurt, egg, and melted butter. Add to the dry ingredients, along with the orange zest, and mix lightly until just combined.

4   Take the baking dish from the oven and dollop the muffin batter on top of the plums, in 8 large spoonfuls to create a rough cobbler effect. Sprinkle a little extra brown sugar over the top.

5   Return the dish to the oven and bake for a further 20–25 minutes or until the muffin topping is golden and cooked. Serve warm with plain yogurt or light sour cream.

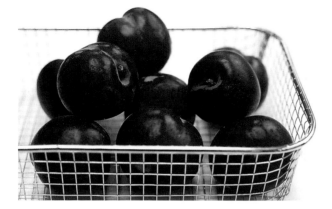

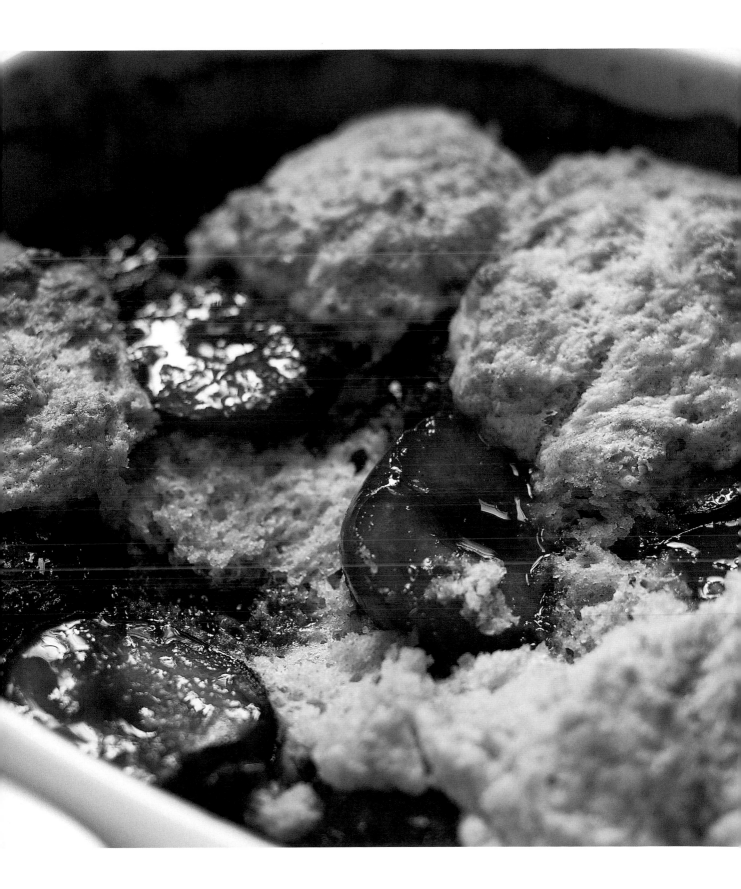

apple and apricot phyllo pie

Phyllo pastry is much lower in fat than other pastries, and you can brush the phyllo layers with milk rather than the more usual melted butter. Here, phyllo envelopes sweet apples and dried apricots to make a crisp, light pie. Serve warm, with crème fraîche or light sour cream.

SERVES 4

4 small tart-sweet apples, cored and sliced
1/2 cup dried apricots, sliced
1/2 teaspoon ground cinnamon
3 tablespoons light brown sugar
grated zest of 1 lemon
squeeze of lemon juice
6 large sheets of phyllo pastry
2 tablespoons milk
1 tablespoon butter, melted
4 tablespoons honey

1 Preheat the oven to 375°F. Toss the apples, dried apricots, cinnamon, brown sugar, and lemon zest and juice together in a large bowl. Set aside.

2 Fold one large sheet of phyllo pastry in half and lay it on a nonstick baking sheet. Brush with a little milk. Cover with another folded sheet of phyllo and brush with milk. Scatter half of the apple and apricot mixture on top.

3 Cover with a further two sheets of folded phyllo, brushing each with milk, then scatter the remaining apple mixture over evenly. Layer the remaining two sheets of phyllo on top, this time brushing with the melted butter.

4 Using a sharp knife, score the top layer of the pie in a diamond pattern. Bake for 40–45 minutes until the apples are cooked and the pastry is golden. Meanwhile, in a saucepan, heat the honey with 4 tablespoons water and simmer for 3 minutes. Set aside to cool slightly.

5 Spoon the honey syrup over the pie and return to the oven for 5 minutes to glaze. Let the pie cool slightly before cutting. Serve warm.

chocolate and raisin brownies

Lowfat cream cheese and naturally sweet raisins make these brownies particularly moist and quite irresistible. They are low in fat, but still taste very chocolatey. They're best eaten on the day of baking.

MAKES 9

$2/3$ cup lowfat cream cheese

$3/4$ cup light brown sugar

$1/2$ cup unsweetened cocoa powder, sifted

2 egg whites

1 teaspoon vanilla extract

1 tablespoon lowfat milk

$1/3$ cup all-purpose flour

$1/2$ teaspoon baking powder

$1/2$ cup raisins

confectioners' sugar, for dusting

1 Preheat the oven to 350°F. Line a 6-inch square baking pan with parchment paper.

2 In a large bowl, combine the cream cheese with the sugar. Add the cocoa powder, egg whites, vanilla extract, and milk. Beat well until the mixture is smooth.

3 Sift the flour and baking powder together over the mixture, then fold in lightly, along with the raisins. Spoon the batter into the prepared pan and bake for 25 minutes until springy to the touch.

4 Remove from the oven and let cool in the pan. Cut into 9 squares and dust the brownies with confectioners' sugar just before serving.

index

Acknowledgements

Firstly my very special thanks to Louise Wooldridge and Jacks Waters for their hard work and dedication, you girls are the best and both deserve medals! I am also very grateful to Janet Illsley, my editor, for all her hard work and advice. Thanks to Gus Filgate, Silvana Franco, Vanessa Courtier, Jane Campsie and Anna-Lisa Aldridge for the brilliant photography. Finally I have to thank Tim, my husband, for always being a devoted taster with a huge appetite.